Praise for *Making the Cut*

"When the courage and integrity of many in the medical community were put to the test, Dr. Aaron Kheriaty passed with flying colors. That so many others failed, reveals that there are broad and deep deficiencies in the culture of medical practice and medical education. In a great many crucial respects, medicine today is in need of healing. In *Making the Cut*, Dr. Kheriaty provides not only diagnosis but also prescription. It is essential reading for anyone interested in how to heal modern medicine."

—**Robert P. George,** McCormick Professor of Jurisprudence at Princeton University and former member of the President's Council on Bioethics

"How is the practice of medicine going to recover from the disaster of 2020 and following? To answer that question comes Dr. Aaron Kheriaty, one of the great heroes of the pandemic period. He reflects on his own early training and growing ambivalence toward professional orthodoxies. His doubts boiled over with the pandemic response that misdiagnosed the disease and cure at multiple levels. Trust has taken a huge hit. The profession must adapt. Dr. Kheriaty's book is a fantastic guide to the healing both we and the practice of medicine desperately need."

—**Jeffrey Tucker,** Founding President of the Brownstone Institute

"This highly readable book is, in part, an account of how and why Aaron Kheriaty survived the rigors of medical school—how he made the cut and became a physician, and why he is grateful for what he regards as the enormous privilege of that calling. But it is also an account of how and why the profession of medicine needs to make the cut—needs, that is, to cut through its enslavement to the managerial and highly centralized approaches that have come to dominate the physician's art. Readers who are drawn in by the first of these, by the personal stories, will in the end find themselves invited to ponder how our approach to medical caregiving might be altered for the better. In the process they may become wiser patients."

—**Gilbert Meilaender,** Senior Research Professor at Valparaiso University

"In the tradition of such medical chronicles as *Intern* and *House of God*, Dr. Kheriaty records his progression from medical student to a full-fledged attending physician by reflecting on the patients he cared for, and who taught him in turn. This outsider, not-quite-orthodox medical student evolves into a questioning physician—and questions abound. Both affectionate critique and pointed criticism from a self-professed reluctant romantic in love with flawed patients and his flawed profession, he looks at his profession as he would a patient and determines that it is sick indeed. This book is his prescription for a cure."

—**G. Kevin Donovan, MD, MA,** Clinical Professor Emeritus and Director of the Center for Clinical Bioethics at Georgetown University

"Aaron Kheriaty has written a modern classic. *Making the Cut* is a captivating memoir cum profound meditation on what ails modern medicine—and how to heal it. Beautifully written, it should be required reading for all doctors and medical students, and really for anyone who cares about the health of our nation and our nation's health."

—**Ryan T. Anderson, PhD,** President of the Ethics and Public Policy Center

"If contemporary medicine has any chance of preserving itself as a coherent practice, the reforms for which Dr. Kheriaty argues here will be at the center of the game plan. Happily, readers will find a book unburdened by dry, hyper-academic, and white-papery prose—but will instead encounter a sophisticated, evidence-based proposal interwoven with and undergirded by Kheriaty's own engrossing story. I cannot wait to use this book in the classroom."

—**Charles Camosy,** bioethicist and author of *Too Expensive to Treat?: Finitude, Tragedy, and the Neonatal ICU*

"In *Making the Cut*, Dr. Aaron Kheriaty offers a luminous and unflinchingly candid memoir that traces the inner contours of medical formation with intellectual rigor and moral clarity. Through richly textured narrative and incisive reflection, he illuminates the ethical complexities, existential inquiries, and quiet crucibles that define the making of a physician. This is a rare work—at once literary and philosophical—that not only bears witness to the hidden struggles and redemptive moments of medical training but also reorients the reader toward the telos of good medicine: the integral flourishing of both patient and healer."

—**Keri O. Brenner, MD, MPA,** Clinical Associate Professor of Medicine at Stanford University

"Everyone knows that navigating the American healthcare system has become a costly nightmare. Perverse incentives mean doctors and hospitals prioritize quick fixes over helping patients achieve long-term health. Fortunately, some doctors are, well, sick of this state of affairs, and Aaron Kheriaty's *Making the Cut* provides a refreshingly humanist dissection of all that's gone wrong, one that seamlessly blends his captivating personal experience as a doctor with eye-opening facts and policy analysis. In the end, Kheriaty demonstrates to readers he's exactly what our health system needs more of—a doctor you can trust."

—**Mollie Hemingway,** Editor in Chief of The Federalist

MAKING THE CUT

How to Heal Modern Medicine

Aaron Kheriaty, MD
Scholar at the Ethics and
Public Policy Center

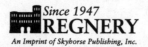

Copyright © 2025 by Aaron Kheriaty

All rights reserved. No part of this book may be reproduced in any manner without the express written consent of the publisher, except in the case of brief excerpts in critical reviews or articles. All inquiries should be addressed to Regnery, 307 West 36th Street, 11th Floor, New York, NY 10018.

Regnery books may be purchased in bulk at special discounts for sales promotion, corporate gifts, fund-raising, or educational purposes. Special editions can also be created to specifications. For details, contact the Special Sales Department, Regnery, 307 West 36th Street, 11th Floor, New York, NY 10018 or info@skyhorsepublishing.com.

Regnery® is an imprint of Skyhorse Publishing, Inc.®, a Delaware corporation.

Visit our website at www.regnery.com.
Please follow our publisher Tony Lyons on Instagram @tonylyonsisuncertain.

10 9 8 7 6 5 4 3 2 1

Library of Congress Cataloging-in-Publication Data is available on file.

Cover design by David Ter-Avanesyan
Cover photograph courtesy of the Ethics and Public Policy Center

Print ISBN: 978-1-5107-8352-2
eBook ISBN: 978-1-5107-8421-5

Printed in the United States of America

For my parents, Larry and Elaine,
without whom I would not have made it to medical school
&
For my wife, Jennifer,
without whom I would not have made it through medical school

CONTENTS

INTRODUCTION
The Reluctant Romantic   1

CHAPTER 1
Into the Breach   13

CHAPTER 2
A Patient Corpse   26

CHAPTER 3
See One, Do One, Teach One   51

CHAPTER 4
Their Exits and Their Entrances   76

CHAPTER 5
Heal with Steel   100

CHAPTER 6
Minds on Fire   122

CHAPTER 7
Only the Trying   133

CHAPTER 8
The Receiving End   153

CHAPTER 9
Quiet Desperation   178

CHAPTER 10
Diagnosing the Disease   196

CHAPTER 11
Making the Cut   218

CONCLUSION
To the Wonder   231

Acknowledgments   245
Notes   247

Author's Note: While all the stories told here are true, the names and other identifying information of patients and other physicians have been altered to protect their privacy.

INTRODUCTION

The Reluctant Romantic

This seeing the sick endears them to us, us too it endears.
—Gerard Manley Hopkins, "Felix Randal"[1]

Some doctors are born with a stethoscope around their neck and a reflex hammer in their crib. They enter medical school by design, and perhaps by destiny. These physicians pass through medical school as a matter of course without questioning—and perhaps without wonder.

I was not one of them.

I progressed through training as a matter of crisis and was continually astonished by what I saw and did. I admit I was not prepared for what training to be a doctor would entail. I took little for granted in medical school, and for some time, I felt like a field anthropologist in some far-off village looking in on a foreign culture and studying the habits of the natives.

When I was young and engaged in the business of wondering what I wanted to be when I grew up, the idea of medicine was often dimly there. But I resisted it. Being a doctor seemed too conventional and quotidian for my aspirations and broad interests. I fancied having a unique or unusual career—not one where I would be melted down and poured into a mold. I hoped to form things, not to be formed, and certainly not to *con*-form. Even when I finally decided to go to medical school, I still saw it as a means to some other, as yet undetermined, end.

But something happened there that I did not expect.

It was not that the powers-that-be broke my will and I fell into lockstep with the other medical lemmings. No, I never lost the sense of being somewhat of a foreigner, a not-quite-orthodox physician. But something in me changed. The spirit of the old Hippocratic physicians—the desire to become a truly skilled and trusted healer—took root in me. "MD" became more than an appendage to my name. The outsider was drawn inside; the skeptic began to believe. Something happened in medical school that should not have surprised me, although it did.

I became a doctor.

This is a story of surprises, for nearly everything during my medical training astonished me. I am embarrassed to admit this now, but I did not have the slightest idea what I was really getting into when I began. I was never the gung-ho pre-med that the toddlers with stethoscopes became in college. It was not just that I never got together with the pre-med crowd in college to watch episodes of *ER*, or that there were no other doctors in my family, or that I decided late in the game that I would pursue a medical degree. Beyond this, my feeling of being an outsider continued through most of my medical training.

Doubts about my decision lingered until my final year. Along the way, I questioned many other things related to the education of physicians and the treatment of patients. Yet I was neither a contrarian who assumed I knew better than my teachers, nor a nonconformist shaking my fist angrily at a flawed system. Mine is a critical, though not a bitter, tale. It is a romance told by a reluctant romantic. I came to medical school prepared to learn, and I learned a great deal about medicine and a great deal about myself. But I also fell in love.

In the end, I became a physician because of the patients I treated. They are the heroes of this book; their stories form the heart of my story. The patients I was privileged to care for during medical school drew this hesitant healer, almost without my realizing it, deeper into the adventure of medicine. Their lives, and their deaths, were the mold into which I was poured. They showed me that, contrary to my expectations, being a physician is anything but conventional, ordinary, or routine.

For this, I thank them.

I first sensed back in medical school that the house of medicine was unwell, though the condition has worsened in the twenty years since then. Without question, as a student, I got to see medicine at its finest. I watched a dogged resident apply every ounce of her intelligence to diagnose an illness so rare that only a few dozen cases had ever been reported. I witnessed a cardiologist shock a man back to life as the patient teetered on the brink of death. I assisted surgeons who replaced dead organs with living ones, giving patients a new lease on life. I saw other doctors after a long day of rounds, surgeries, and clinic stick around to console a dying woman or counsel a young man who only narrowly escaped death by drug overdose.

I also saw strange and awful sights I could not have previously imagined: a liquified brain in an anatomy dissection lab, cockroaches scurrying across the hospital floor, a young man who deliberately swallowed a razor and lit himself on fire, a mute priest wasting away and wracked with pain, a female surgeon barely five feet tall who was rumored to throw surgical instruments at hapless residents in the operating room, a mysterious patient who escaped for the briefest moment from the silent prison of his broken brain, and a man who wanted to give his kidney to a perfect stranger.

But there's a downside to seeing something done well, because then you know what it means to fall short of that standard. See medicine practiced beautifully and you know what it means for it to get ugly. You can only diagnose disease if you have a sense of what *health* looks like. At medical school, I was lucky enough to see medicine at its finest, but that vision only served to amplify its serious failures.

I'd secured admission to one of the best medical schools in the country. Looking back, I must confess to having donned an unearned swagger—at least at the beginning. I sauntered onto the streets of

Georgetown like so many unattractive overachievers. But I wasn't just overconfident. Worse, if I'm honest, I just didn't think it was going to be that difficult. I was smart. I was arrogant. And I was completely wrong.

Getting through medical school proved far more difficult than getting in. Making the cut was an ordeal. It meant digesting enormous quantities of information (275 diseases in pathology, 276 medications in pharmacology, 206 bones and 900 ligaments among thousands of structures in anatomy, and on and on), navigating a complex but unspoken hospital hierarchy (*How long do I wait before I page the attending a second time?*), steadying sweaty hands while performing my first lumbar puncture on an unsuspecting patient, and mastering the foreign languages of medical jargon and hospital slang. My first glance at a patient's chart on the wards required translating this acronymic fever dream that no medical textbook had prepared me for: "59 y.o. WM č h/o CAD, HTN, ^chol & CHF, s/p CABG x 4, presents ER c 4/10 CP rad LUE x 3h, š n/v/f/c/s . . ."

> The patient is a fifty-nine-year-old white male with a history of coronary artery disease, hypertension, hypercholesterolemia, and congestive heart failure; status: post four-vessel coronary artery bypass graft, who presents to the emergency room with chest pain radiating to the left upper extremity for the past three hours, which is four out of ten on a scale of intensity, without any associated nausea, vomiting, fever, chills, or sweats.

I was naïvely unaware when I entered medical school that my duties would include manually disimpacting an almost 500-pound, severely constipated man who screamed in agony for his mother—despite the fact that we loaded him with morphine prior to this gruesome procedure—while we dug hard, reeking stool from his rectum. All in a day's work.

Becoming a doctor took more than completing courses and passing exams. It meant accompanying patients and their families through incredible anguish and loss. The physical strain of sleep deprivation and thirty-six-hour shifts was benign in comparison to these challenges. How do I explain to a woman with a four-year-old son that's barely hanging on to life in our pediatric intensive care unit that her other teenage son was just admitted to the psychiatry ward in the same hospital and diagnosed with his first psychotic break after jumping out of a moving car? How do we help a family understand that their loved one is not a candidate for a life-saving organ transplant they had been waiting for? How do I say goodbye to someone we couldn't save?

I often doubted that I would make the cut. During my second year, I wavered between sticking it out or calling it quits. Had I known what I was getting into, I never would have embarked upon medical school. But when it was over, and only then—paradoxically—I stopped being able to imagine doing anything else. It seems that I did not choose medicine. It chose me.

When I was accepted to medical school, I did not fully realize how fortunate I was to have been given a spot. With thousands of superb applicants turned down each year, I had won the lottery. Sure, I had studied hard, but everyone had studied hard.

The problem was that I thought medical school would be straightforward. I thought my previous academic success had prepared me to excel in this new arena. But I quickly learned that this isn't how med school works. Not at all, as you will see in these pages.

To this day, I remain both an insider and an outsider to medicine—a grateful practitioner and concerned critic. For sixteen years following residency, I rose through the ranks of academic medicine at the University of California, Irvine, as a professor in the School of Medicine and the director of the hospital's Medical Ethics Program.

Three times I was honored with the Excellence in Teaching Award from medical students. I planned to stay at the university until retirement, enjoying a prestigious and rewarding career in academic medicine, firmly ensconced within the medical establishment.

But when I perceived the institution was losing its ethical bearings during the Covid crisis, I decided to challenge its misguided vaccine mandate policy in federal court. In retaliation, I quickly found myself out of a job and banished from campus. But not once have I regretted my decision.

Not long after that, when my state passed a law restricting the free speech rights of physicians—California's ill-fated Assembly Bill 2098—I again went to federal court with four fellow physician plaintiffs to challenge the law. A physician with a gag order is not a doctor you can trust, and I was convinced this misguided law was disastrous for both physicians and patients. We filed a suit called *Hoeg v. Newsom* and obtained a preliminary injunction against the unconstitutional law. Seeing that the law would surely be defeated in court, the state legislature then repealed it.

The following year, when we discovered the federal government had been censoring the speech of credible doctors and scientists on social media, in clear violation of our free speech rights, I once again pushed back. I filed a First Amendment challenge, along with the states of Missouri and Louisiana and four other private plaintiffs, in federal court. We took the case, *Missouri v. Biden*, all the way to the US Supreme Court. The federal district court judge, in granting our petition for a preliminary injunction against the government on July 4, 2023, said that this was "arguably the worst violation of free speech in United States history."[2]

When I see medicine losing its way, when I see policymakers pushing medicine and public health in destructive directions, I am not someone who can stand idly on the sidelines. I diagnose and attempt to treat the serious problems in contemporary medicine out of a sense of personal heartbreak for something I love dearly—for a noble profession that has been recklessly squandering the public's trust and abandoning our mandate to heal.

This book is about the art of healing and the dangers that threaten it. Medicine is an ancient profession that has made astonishing advances in recent history. Who among us wants to return to the days of the Civil War, when surgeons amputated gangrenous legs and removed cancerous breasts without anesthesia? Who wants a world without antibiotics, even if these wonder drugs are now becoming less effective by the year, breeding treatment-resistant bugs through overuse?

Nobody wants a world without ventilators and dialysis machines, which can maintain life after organs fail, even if too many unfortunate souls are consigned by modern medicine to a bare biological life, permanently tethered to these organ-replacement technologies. Modern medicine may be a mixed blessing, but it is a blessing.

For all its impressive advances, however, medicine still meets with only modest success and appears to be getting diminishing returns despite technological innovations. We cure more cancers, but we contract more cancers. We live longer, but with more years of chronic decline and disability. Many diseases—from muscular dystrophy to Alzheimer's to autism—remain largely outside the ken of science and beyond the healing powers of doctors. We know that many medications work, but we often have no idea *how* they work. And all of them come with downstream costs. Medicine often claims knowledge and powers it does not actually possess, and much of the public is more than willing to play along. But more people today are waking up to these facts, questioning our healthcare system, and doubting conventional wisdom in medicine.

The early-twentieth-century writer G. K. Chesterton was fond of saying, "If a thing is worth doing, it is worth doing badly."[3] This might sound strange, indulgent even—like it is rationalizing mediocrity.

After all, when life hangs in the balance, why should doctors accept doing medicine "badly"? Yet this sense of never feeling up to the task and still pressing ahead lies at the heart of medicine. The recurring experience of those who treat the sick is this: One never quite feels adequate. For every patient we save with a ruptured aortic aneurism, like the one I treated on my penultimate day of medical school, there are dozens more who never make it to the hospital or who die on the operating table.

Nevertheless, doctors must still try to stem the tide of suffering and illness, even when the results appear meager. "People not only expect of [the physician] what he can do but what he cannot do," psychiatrist and philosopher Karl Jaspers said in his essay "The Idea of the Physician." "The world asks him for every kind of help, and it wants more. . . . For all his triumphs, the physician feels more strongly what he cannot do than what he can."[4]

Consider what the doctor is up against. Disease has been a permanent feature of human life from the beginning, and it shows few signs of abating—the vaunted miracles of modern medicine notwithstanding. Contrary to the blank checks that some overzealous geneticists and transhumanists are writing, the last "enemy," death, will never be conquered by science and technology. Life is a sexually transmitted condition that is invariably fatal. And it always will be: The human mortality rate continues to hold steady at 100 percent. As Cormac McCarthy said of a gangster in his novel *No Country for Old Men*, "He died of natural causes. Natural to the line of work he was in. . . ."[5]

As if the natural enemies we face—disease, disability, death—aren't threatening enough, the physician also contends with the works of mankind: war, terror, violence in our streets. And stupidity. An emergency physician once told me most of the patients he sees end up in the ER because the patient did something idiotic—often involving guns, self-injury, or objects jammed into various bodily orifices (ah, dear reader, the X-rays I could show you. . .).

While I was in medical school, a band of malicious men with a few knives and plane tickets were able to fill the hospitals and morgues of Manhattan and Washington, DC, on September 11, 2001. What are our efforts worth in the face of such malice? And yet, the physician still believes it's worthwhile . . . if only he can spare this one life, this one desperate person who is lying helpless and vulnerable in front of him.

Despite his impotence, and despite his inadequacy, when facing the slings and arrows of outrageous fortune, suffering, ugliness, pain, and death, the physician soldiers on. This does not mean that he wears blinders. The physician remains acutely aware of human frailty and folly. Nonetheless, as Jaspers added, "He binds up small wounds while other men keep striking larger ones."[6] Being a doctor is often about embracing futility—while forgetting that's what you're doing. It's about winning provisional battles in a long war that is already lost.

How does one prepare for this task? How does one become proficient in the art of healing—even when all cures remain at best only temporary? How does one train for a job where success inevitably involves huge doses of failure? Medical school is an exceptional training ground, unlike anything else in the professional world. During my medical training, I was permitted to do things that in any other context would have been considered a felony: like carving up a dead body or practicing unperfected procedural skills on unsuspecting patients.

This book's setting—the modern hospital and clinic, with its high-tech wizardry and human life-and-death drama—is an intriguing world unto itself. Television producers seem to have discovered that hospitals provide at least as much fodder for weekly drama as do courtrooms and cops on the beat. People outside of medicine want to hear what it is like to dissect a dead body, to comfort a dying patient, to save a life after a trauma, to encounter a psychotic and mentally ill patient, to assist in performing surgery on an eyeball, to watch the West Nile Virus take someone overnight from a healthy to delirious state and then to the grave, to deliver a baby and then place him in the arms of his mother.

When our medical institutions are compromised by money, power, or other interests external to healing the sick, and when medical schools succumb to ideological fads, the risks to individuals and society cannot be overstated. If medicine itself is sick, we are all in trouble. Ignoring the illness only allows it to metastasize. That is why I have written this book.

The story I tell here is a brief chapter in the history of medicine—a story which is very old. A student once asked the famous anthropologist Margaret Mead a fascinating question: "What is the earliest sign of human civilization we have discovered?" The student probably expected her to say something like a piece of pottery or perhaps a fragment of a handheld tool. But Mead replied that the first sign of human civilization was a healed femur—a fifteen-thousand-year-old human thigh bone.[7]

In a primitive society, a person with a broken leg would have nothing to contribute to the functioning of the community. The injured patient was only a drain on the collective resources, a group liability. After the bone was set by someone in the tribe who possessed the requisite skill, and while it slowly healed, the injured person would have to be carried from place to place, fed, sheltered, and tended to for months—without any ability to contribute to the survival of the community. *And yet this person did live long enough for the broken leg to heal.* This means that he was cared for by a knowledgeable healer and supported collectively by his entire community, even at considerable cost and at some risk to the welfare of the others. This was the first sign of a civilized society.

When I am tempted to become cynical about the future of medicine, I find it helpful to recall that this venerable practice of healing the sick signals the very dawn of civilization. Contrary to popular belief, perhaps medicine is the oldest profession.

Somewhere along the way, however, medicine got sick. A recent survey of almost half a million Americans published in the *Journal of the American Medical Association* showed that trust in physicians and hospitals plummeted during the Covid crisis, from 72 percent in 2020 to 40 percent in 2024. Four themes emerged to account for this waning trust: financial motives over patient care, poor quality of care and negligence, undue influence of external agencies and agendas, and concerns about discrimination and bias.[8] Another recent post-Covid Pew Research Center survey likewise found that 71 percent of Americans doubt medical scientists will act in the best interest of the public, a ten-point increase compared to a few years prior.[9]

Meanwhile, we are grappling with an epidemic of chronic illness—heart disease, cancer, diabetes, obesity, metabolic syndrome, Alzheimer's, stroke, and chronic lung and kidney disease—affecting six in ten Americans, which medicine seems powerless to fix.[10] Starting in 2014, the overall life expectancy of Americans has declined for the first time since the 1918 influenza pandemic, according to a report from the National Academies of Sciences, Engineering, and Medicine.[11] We spend twice as much on healthcare per capita than any other country but barely rank in the top fifty in terms of health outcomes. As I will explore in later chapters, like the old Soviet Union, the US healthcare system has evolved so that a whole bunch of vested interests can extract rents from a bloated, dysfunctional bureaucracy. But patients are left to suffer.

Not only are trust levels tanking and diseases worsening, but the number of doctors also is dropping dramatically. Physicians are quitting in droves. According to the American Medical Association, one in five doctors will leave medicine in the next two years, while one in three will reduce their hours.[12] "You're not just burned out," my colleagues in medicine tell me. "You've been abused." Physicians are more likely to die by suicide than other professionals and the general population, according to a report from the *General Hospital Psychiatry* journal.[13]

A doctor, we assume, wounds in order to heal. "You're going to feel a sharp pain!" she says, before making the cut. But today, the doctor all too often wounds *without* healing. Why?

This idea of doctors *causing* sickness—so-called "iatrogenic disease" (now the fifth leading cause of death worldwide)—evokes images of medieval physicians applying leeches to the skin to suck out the patient's blood. In fact, in middle English "lece" meant both *doctor* and *leech*! Modern medicine still harbors its own insidious leeches—personnel and institutional forces that capitalize on our sickness while further sucking out our life and health.

Sad to say, the highest aim of modern medicine is not health, but rather efficiency. Today, medicine has often become more adept at controlling bodies than curing them. Like other fields, it has fatally succumbed to managerialism—the quixotic belief that, through the accumulation of "rational" knowledge, everything can and should be engineered and managed from the top down. This ignores the fact that every patient is unique and therefore should not be "processed" through an industrial-scale, people-moving turnstile medical system that treats every patient exactly the same.

The word *crisis* in English (from the Greek *krises*—"decision") was originally a medical term denoting a disease's critical turning point, the moment we know whether someone will recover or die. Safe to say, then, that modern medicine is in crisis.

I do think there's a cure for medicine's ills, but it's going to hurt. Effective treatment, as every doctor knows, begins with an accurate diagnosis. Before asking Vladimir Lenin's question, "What is to be done?" we must ask Marvin Gaye's, "What's going on?" This book is about what's going on in the house of medicine and how we might begin to fix it.

This is also the story of how I changed during the course of my medical training. It's about what medicine gave me—and what it sometimes took from me. It's about how I grew from an overconfident pre-med to an ambivalent medical student to a capable physician who had fallen in love with medicine—even if my lover has turned into a prostitute of late. While this book presents a sharply critical diagnosis of contemporary medicine, I apply the wounding scalpel in order to heal.

CHAPTER 1

Into the Breach

If blood will flow when flesh and steel are one
Drying in the colour of the evening sun
Tomorrow's rain will wash the stains away
But something in our minds will always stay
—Sting, "Fragile"[1]

The patient was literally full of shit.

It was our job to remedy this. We were certainly trying. But now our forty-year-old patient, I'll call him Mr. Dolor, was screaming—I mean *really* screaming—in anguish, calling out for his mother. "Mama! Ahhhh! *MAMA! OWWW!*" he shrieked in agony. The stench was overpowering. I'll explain why in a moment.

Mr. Dolor was an enormous mountain of flesh, weighing in at nearly five hundred pounds. He was entirely bedridden due to his girth, taking opiates for pain, and now hospitalized on our service. The combination of his sedentary ways and the gut-stopping pain meds meant that he had not had a bowel movement in several weeks. The previous medical team had failed to monitor this, and now it was our problem.

The abdominal X-ray showed massive amounts of stool stuck in his grossly distended, functionally paralyzed colon. Mr. Dolor's constipation was so severe that he could no longer take food or water by mouth; he would immediately vomit, his gastrointestinal system rejecting anything that landed in the stomach. Fortunately, he did not require much nutrition because he had plenty of reserves. But this could not go on forever.

Constipation is a common problem in hospitals. Mild forms can be resolved "from above" using oral remedies from laxatives to stool softeners. More severe forms require unplugging the system "from below" with rectal suppositories or an enema. We had tried everything for Mr. Dolor with remedies from both directions, all to no avail.

Well . . . almost everything.

"It's time for the last resort," the resident informed me. "Come on, we need to go manually disimpact him." We physicians have the most anodyne terms for procedures.

Poor Mr. Dolor lay on his side, gripping the rails of his hospital bed. We loaded him with a generous dose of morphine even though it might slow his bowels further; he would need some palliation for this procedure. I'm not sure the morphine did any good. To his credit, the senior resident did not pawn this task off on the intern but snapped on the gloves himself—double gloves for this one. He stuck out his fingers, and I applied the lubricant generously, recalling the sage advice from the stand-in patient-actor who taught me how to do the rectal exam: "You can never have too much lubricant." Sound advice indeed. People from the local community volunteer for this instructional role so that a medical student's first rectal or pelvic exam is not practiced on an actual patient. My tattooed and grizzled volunteer looked like he had driven there on his Harley, and I never forgot his word of advice.

"Here goes," the resident said, holding up his lubricated finger. "You'll feel a bit of pressure," he informed Mr. Dolor with a bedside euphemism almost cruel in its studied understatement. My job was to separate and hold Mr. Dolor's butt cheeks apart so that the resident could gain access to his anus. The resident inserted one finger and dug out a glop of hard, reeking stool. Mr. Dolor's wailing commenced.

Undeterred, the resident continued—into the breach once more. In time, he escalated to two fingers. The reek was almost unbearable. I suppressed a wretch, tasting the vomit in the back of my throat and swallowing hard. My hands continued to separate Mr. Dolor's enormous glutes, though my arms were growing tired, and I was beginning to perspire. Standing to the side of the resident, I lacked the proper angle to get sufficient leverage. Medical school is 10 percent smarts and 90 percent grit, I reminded myself.

The resident kept digging, and the foul excrement kept emerging. The patient's screams did not cease until we were finished. Afterwards, whimpering a bit, Mr. Dolor actually thanked us and apologized for the unpleasantness.

"No problem," I said, patting him on the shoulder, "that's why we're here."

Granted, it's not what idealistic pre-med undergraduates dream about. I'll admit that it's not the scene I imagined when I entered medical school. But very little about medical school turned out to fit my prior expectations. By my final year of training, I was not shocked to find myself assisting with this manual disimpaction procedure—for the entire four years had been a parade of surprises.

Real medicine is rarely sexy. Sometimes it's plain gross. Doctors do what needs to be done. We reach into the biological muck when others recoil, as firefighters run into burning buildings when sane people flee the flames. Is medicine's beauty to be found precisely in its ugliness? Can medicine extract treasures from the bodily mess of bones and blood and bile? Were we merely shoveling shit that day, or healing the world one morbidly constipated patient at a time? Was this succor or torture? Were we only wounding, or wounding to heal?

Whatever the answers, I wish for Mr. Dolor's sake that we could have done the damnable deed under anesthesia. Or at least with his mother at the bedside to hold his hand.

Stiffen the sinews, summon up the blood. Once more into the breach. One last time.

"They're bringing him by helicopter . . . it's a ruptured triple-A coming in tonight," the surgery resident, Juan, informed me, a gleam in his eye. "You want to stick around for it?"

In fewer than twenty-four hours, I would be finished with medical school. I had been counting the weeks, then the days, and now the hours. That day, I'd been up since 4:30 a.m. and had already worked fourteen hours. So the prospect of "sticking around for it" was not appealing. I wanted to get home and see my wife, Jennifer, and our two-year-old son, John. I had every right to decline, and every reason. Yet I found myself hesitating.

"Sure, I'll stay. Let me call my wife."

The resident smiled. "The chopper is on its way. Should be here in less than an hour . . ."

Why did I decide to stick around? I don't really know. I no longer needed to make an impression, having already "matched" at my residency program of choice and signed my contract (finally, a modest paycheck!). The surgery grade didn't matter. (Even if it did, leaving at 6:00 p.m. rather than 12:00 a.m. on the penultimate day wouldn't have adversely impacted my grade anyway). Nor was I motivated by the prospect of more surgical training. I was not destined for surgery.

I guess it was this, then: Ultimately, I wanted to finish on a high. I wanted to go out not with a whimper but with a bang. And from what I'd heard, choppering towards me was a real banger of a case.

I collapsed in the residents' workroom, piled some cold Indian food onto a paper plate—courtesy of a pharma rep, always eager to bribe us with food—and began fueling up for the late night.

Meanwhile, flying by helicopter from West Virginia to Washington, DC, was a fifty-nine-year-old man who, until a few hours ago, had been going about his usual business blithely unaware of the time-bomb about to explode in his belly. Even now, thanks to the sedatives, he remained blissfully ignorant of his dire condition. He was resting serenely with a breathing tube in his throat. Medications to strengthen the contractions of his heart were being infused by IV. His feet were turning blue.

A "triple-A," or "abdominal aortic aneurysm," is often a silent killer. It involves a rupture in the largest blood vessel in the body. The aorta—weakened from years of chronic metabolic ills—blows up slowly, until one day the wall becomes too thin for the pressure inside, and the vessel pops like an overinflated balloon. This results in sudden massive bleeding into the abdominal cavity. Until a rupture occurs, someone with a triple-A can be completely without subjective symptoms, and like the man in the helicopter, entirely unaware of the deadly ticking time-bomb in his belly.

Almost all patients who rupture the aorta bleed to death internally, typically within minutes, before help can arrive. But if you're lucky enough—as this man was—to have the rupture occur toward the back of the vessel, the bleeding may become walled-off by surrounding structures, buying him perhaps a few precious hours that could be long enough for us to cut open his abdomen and clamp the bleeding aorta in time. According to the brief report we received from the rural emergency room where he had presented, the patient's blood pressure was dropping, his heart rate was escalating, and his "mental status" was tending toward delirium. All clear signs of hemorrhagic shock.

The patient was dying. The clock was ticking. We were waiting.

"This is what it's all about!" Juan exclaimed. Some people are born to wield a scalpel, like this Colombian-born resident on call that night. "All this residency training . . . five years of this crap. This is where it all pays off," he said with a gleam in his eye.

We were walking down the hall, still waiting for the chopper to arrive. Juan debriefed me on the basics of this surgery before shooting off down the hall again, walking at a breakneck surgery resident's pace. "When I page you to '111,' meet me on the helicopter pad."

"Where's the helicopter pad?" I shot back. But he had already disappeared around the corner. Like most things in medical school, I'd have to figure this out myself.

Today's doctors are at their best when dealing with disasters. An acute life-threatening emergency, like this triple-A, displays the virtues of modern medicine in living color. Contemporary medicine is better at emergency intervention than sustained assistance, much less preventive care. Why? Because the reductionistic philosophy which shapes modern medicine inclines physicians to see the body as a broken machine in need of repair, rather than an impaired organic whole in need of nurturing. Granted, sometimes the body does look something like a broken machine, as in this case of a ruptured aneurism. The engine has blown a gasket, and the doctor must open the hood, reach inside with his tools, and fix it before everything collapses.

But this is only a limited and partial view of health and illness. Historian of medicine E. Richard Brown argued that this mechanistic view gained dominance in medicine not because it is the most accurate account of nature, but because it was congenial to the class of influential modern industrialists in the early twentieth century: "The precise analysis of the human body into its component parts is analogous to the industrial organization of production. From the perspective of an industrialist, scientific medicine seems to offer the limitless potential for effectiveness that science and technology provide in manufacturing and social organization." This view of the body assumed that "just as industry depends upon science for technically powerful industrial tools, science-based medicine and its mechanistic concepts of the body and disease should yield powerful tools with which to identify, eliminate, and prevent agents of disease and to correct malfunctions of the body."[2] With this view, health becomes merely the absence of disease, while medicine becomes an engineering task of understanding and manipulating the body's component parts. This philosophy of medicine also tends to encourage a fetish with novel technologies of control—mRNA vaccines, for example—that can introduce considerable risks, while neglecting time-tested remedies simply because they are old.

But industrialized medicine is largely failing to deliver on this promise, often causing more harm than healing, as we will continue to explore further. The mechanistic understanding of health and disease—the view of the body as a machine or manufacturing plant—has dominated medicine for over a century. While serving as a powerful metaphor, it largely blinds us to the real needs of the healthy or sick organism.

Given these mechanistic underpinnings of modern medicine, the ideal doctor today is the trauma surgeon—a detached technician who splices open the battered body to clamp, transfuse, suture, splint, medicate, and shock the patient back to life. The best training ground for trauma surgery is a war zone, with the next best setting an inner-city hospital like Bellevue in New York City or Los Angeles General Medical Center, which often mirrors a war zone. Modern medicine is great for repairing gunshot wounds, stab injuries, blunt force trauma from car crashes, broken bones, acute appendicitis, and ruptured aortas. If, God forbid, you are ever assaulted by a psychopath or run over by a truck, you'll appreciate what our medical system can do—applying impressive technological wizardry and human ingenuity to repair broken arteries and rebuild shattered bones.

However, modern medicine falters when treating chronic conditions, often making them worse. If the aorta ruptures, go to the hospital. But to prevent the chronic conditions that led to an aneurism in the first place—from hypertension to metabolic syndrome—medicine today fights losing battles with mostly ineffective tools. We are facing an epidemic of chronic illnesses, which almost appears to be by design. After all, medicine profits when patients remain sick and endlessly tethered to our expensive "healthcare" system.[3]

In a Goldman Sachs biotech research report in 2018, investment analysts said the quiet part out loud when they asked openly, "Is curing patients a sustainable business model?" They admitted that single-treatment cures are bad for business in the long run because they deprive pharmaceutical companies of recurrent revenue: "While this proposition [curing disease] carries tremendous value for patients and society, it could represent a challenge for genome medicine developers looking for sustained cash flow."[4]

These chronic diseases constitute the leading causes of death and disability in the United States and are leading drivers of the nation's $4.5 trillion in annual healthcare costs. We're great at inserting plates and screws to align broken bones. We're not so great at treating obesity, autism, chronic pain, metabolic derangements, or schizophrenia. Cultivating long-term health is less like "doing battle" with an enemy called disease (how medicine typically sees itself) and more like patiently cultivating a garden where the human body can flourish (here, medicine lacks the resources and the requisite philosophy).

But I'm getting ahead of myself. Before critiquing medicine's manifest shortcomings, I should acknowledge its extraordinary triumphs—like the one we had during my last night of medical school.

"Are you doing anything?" The intern on call, not a member of my vascular surgery team, wasn't supposed to assign me work. Especially *his* work.

"Yeah, we've got a ruptured triple-A on the way."

"He's not here yet, is he? Can you scrub in on Dr. Rosales's case for me? I got a patient who's bradycardic on the floor. I'm supposed to help Rosales, but I've got to take care of this guy first."

"Well . . . uh, the triple-A is on his way. I don't want to miss it." I could see it now: I stick around to see something exciting only to end up covering for the intern. I had no desire to hold retractors—the med student's typical job in the OR, keeping the surgical wound open—for another routine surgery that night.

"Don't worry. I'll scrub you out in ten minutes. This won't take long."

I reluctantly agreed.

The intern kept his word: I only stayed with Rosales's case a few minutes before the intern came to relieve me of duty. Shortly after tearing off my surgical mask and walking out, I got the page from Juan: "111." Here we go, I thought. Up to the helipad. Under my breath, I muttered a Hail Mary for the patient: *Please, God, let him live.* And, in good medical student fashion, I added: *And let me not screw anything up.*

As a medical student, "surgery" is typically limited to holding retractors, cutting sutures, suctioning body fluids out of the surgical field, and sewing up or stapling skin. I had been allowed to cut tissue once, only to be informed afterwards that the department chair wouldn't have approved of a student wielding the scalpel. But however insignificant, I still had a role, especially on the triple-A case. After all, they would need to see the vessel to clamp it, and it is impossible for an attending surgeon to see a bleeding vessel without adequate suction and retraction. I too would have blood on my gloves and sweat on my brow.

I punched in the code on the keypad, and the automatic doors to the helipad swung open. The patient was just then being taken down from the helicopter, lying strapped to a gurney. Juan was already there.

"Hold this," he said, handing me a CT scan from the other emergency room. "Make sure we have it in the OR."

I placed the scan on the gurney next to the patient and began helping to wheel the patient to the elevator. I pressed the down button, felt the elevator drop, then stop, the doors still closed, then . . . we were going *up*. The doors opened to the same floor.

"What the . . . ?" Juan shouted as he jammed his finger repeatedly into the down button. Not an ideal time for an elevator malfunction. The second time around, we dropped, the door opened to the correct floor, and we pushed the patient hurriedly to the operating room.

"Go tell Dr. Rosales the patient's here," Juan commanded. "He's in OR 9. We're in 12." I know, I was just in there, I thought. I refastened my surgical mask and pinched the flexible metal piece over my nose.

The operating room was buzzing. When it's time for action, surgical trauma bays and ORs feel charged, like the air outside during an electrical storm. In this taut atmosphere, an experienced surgeon conducts the symphony of players surrounding the patient—anesthesiologist, nurse, tech, resident, med student—channeling our urgency and energy into precise, focused, elegantly coordinated action. You get the sense that at any moment the situation may collapse into chaos. *If something goes sideways, will things unravel?* You hope there are no technical—or human—glitches in the system: no malfunctioning elevators, no slips of the scalpel.

Within seconds, we transferred the patient to the operating table. The anesthesiologist worked quickly. Already intubated and fully loaded with multiple large-bore intravenous lines, the patient was anesthetized within two minutes.

"Get me a razor," Juan ordered, but before I could find one, he had changed his mind—there was no time to shave the hair off the patient's belly. Juan was furiously "prepping" the patient, scrubbing the abdomen with brown betadine disinfectant solution and rapidly arranging sterile blue drapes around the surgical field.

I hustled out of the room to the scrub station to slather my arms with betadine wash. Normally, one is supposed to take one's time doing this, thoroughly and carefully sponging fingernails to elbows. But this was no time for excess scrubbing and the subtle niceties of perfect infection control. The patient was on the table bleeding to death. My arms and hands were clean enough to do the job.

I raced back into the OR and pivoted to open the door by pushing with my back so that my hands would not be contaminated, arms raised and dripping. "Sterile towel, please. Thanks." A nurse held up my sterile gown so I could slip it on without touching the outside, then she held up my size eight gloves, first right, then left. *Snap. Snap.* Ready.

"Aaron, you here?" For some reason, Dr. Rosales had taken a liking to me over the past month. He seemed glad I was scrubbed in on this case. I was glad he was glad.

"Right here, sir."

I made my way to the attending's side at the operating table. Juan was already making the incision with a scalpel, straight down the middle of the abdomen, from sternum to pelvic bone. I picked up the suction, anticipating a gush of blood when Juan pierced the abdominal cavity. I was not disappointed. I had never seen so much blood. The patient was still alive . . . just barely. "Anesthesia? What's his blood pressure?" Dr. Rosales was grabbing loops of small intestine, pulling them out of the belly to get the patient's guts out of the way. We clamped retractors in place to keep his abdominal cavity splayed open. More suction, and still more blood. Liters of precious red fluid. Juan dug his hand behind the intestines, searching for the ruptured aorta. The blood kept coming faster than I could suction it away.

"I've got my fingers on it—large clamp!" He swiped the clamp from the nurse's hand, inserted it in place blindly, and snapped it shut. More suction. The bleeding had slowed. "Iliac clamps," Juan ordered. "What's his pressure?"

We were sweating and breathing heavily. But the patient was no longer bleeding heavily. We tied off the small bleeding branches of the aorta with sutures. Then we could work more slowly. Seven minutes was all it took from the moment of incision to full control of all the bleeding. It felt like seconds.

The surgical attending and resident performed a clean aortic repair, put the patient's guts back into the abdomen, and closed the deep connective tissue with thick sutures. Then I stapled the skin shut. Blood pressure: 126 over 85.

He had survived. Sweet, sweet success.

In those intense moments, I remember seeing, resting on the patient's chest, his small intestine. His guts were held there by a clamp and a sterile towel. Slowly, with rhythmic wavelike movements, the smooth muscles of the intestine were still contracting in an involuntary motion called "peristalsis," while his chest underneath rose and fell to the rhythm of the respirator settings. Even there, anesthetized on the operating table, his lifeblood draining away, this patient continued to move food through his gut. Yesterday's lunch was traversing . . . over his chest. I smiled at the surreal strangeness of it all.

Minutes later, physically exhausted and emotionally drained, I wheeled the patient up to the intensive care unit. He was still intubated and would likely not wake up for some time. I never saw him conscious, never spoke a word to him. The only feature of his that I remember was that he looked older than his stated age.

"Is this the triple-A, bed 8?" the charge nurse asked me.

"Yes."

"You know anything about this patient?" the ICU physician questioned.

I rehearsed the minimal history that had been sent over from the rural hospital. The patient was a fifty-nine-year-old male with a past medical history significant only for hypertension and high cholesterol. No known drug allergies, taking aspirin, Lipitor, and Cozaar. His symptoms had started at 4:00 p.m. with sudden-onset lower abdominal pain . . .

The physician nodded as I rehearsed the remainder of the patient's history and the course of his surgery.

Midnight. Time for a few hours of sleep. Only one day remaining.

After rounds the next morning, Juan turned to me and said, "Go home, Aaron."

"What?"

"You did a good job here. Go home. Take your kid to the park. Enjoy your time off before residency starts. The next few weeks are the only time in your life when you're an MD with absolutely no clinical responsibilities. Live it up."

I was not expecting this. "Thanks, man!" I was so ecstatic to leave the hospital that I forgot to go through the bureaucratic checkout procedures: turning in my ID badge, pager, library card, and intranet codes. I made a quick stop to pick up flowers for my wife and a bottle of champagne before heading home. I hoped Jennifer and John would be there when I arrived with the news.

"What are you doing here?" Jennifer looked up expectantly, surprised to see me home so early.

"We did it," I smiled. "I'm a doctor."

This is the story of how I got there and what I have learned since then.

CHAPTER 2

A Patient Corpse

Questions of science, science and progress
Do not speak as loud as my heart
—Coldplay, "The Scientist"[1]

"Hello," my father said, answering the phone.
"Hello, is this Mr. Kheriaty?"
"Yes."
"How would you like to go to medical school?"
"Well, I wouldn't. But my son might. This is Aaron's father."
"Oh, I apologize. I'm calling from the University of Pittsburgh to inform you that Aaron has been accepted here." Too late. I had been on the waiting list at Pitt but had not heard from them all summer. By this time, medical school was scheduled to start in a few days. In one whirlwind summer, I had graduated from college, married my high school sweetheart, taken a brief honeymoon, moved cross-country, and settled into a small basement apartment in Washington, DC. Georgetown University School of Medicine would be my home for the next four years.

The decision to attend Georgetown had not been difficult. Prior to my late news from Pittsburgh, only two medical schools had accepted me. The other school had worried my wife when we visited, located as it was in a rather rough neighborhood of Chicago. By contrast, we fell in love with DC; the neighborhood around Georgetown, its row houses, parks, and the nearby museums and cultural attractions were charming and inviting. I was also impressed by the school's tradition and strong reputation.

My first medical school interview had been at the University of Washington in my home state. Since I was a state resident, tuition there would have been about one-sixth the cost of a private or out-of-state medical education. Although I appeared to have the grades and numbers for acceptance to this school, the interview had gone sour. I differed from the interviewers in my position on abortion. Most of the interview consisted of a barrage of questions aimed at hammering out my views on the subject. The guidebooks for medical school interviews will tell you not to worry because they are not supposed to ask questions about ethics, politics, or religion—or if they do, they will not hold it against you if they disagree. That turned out not to be true.

Georgetown students officially begin medical school with what they call the "White Coat Ceremony." It was a rather officious affair, well staged and surprisingly stirring. We sat in Georgetown's majestic Gaston Hall and listened to the eminent ethicist and physician Dr. Edmund Pellegrino, who later became my mentor, give an inspiring speech about the philosophy of medicine.[2] He spoke to us, the initiates into this venerable profession, about the significance of taking the Hippocratic Oath. His remarks that day echoed themes from his ethical writings about medicine as a way of life: "Ethics is more than the application of prima facie principles to specific cases. It is also an invitation to a way of life, to the complete formation of the human person. In medicine, ethics not only resolves dilemmas; it also has the positive function of so ordering the process of healing and decision making as to enhance the humanity of the sick person and of the health worker as well."[3]

In modern usage, we have become accustomed to calling just about any occupation a "profession," but this was not customary in the ancient world. For the Greeks and Romans, the term *profession* was used to designate only four occupations: medicine, law, teaching, and the priesthood. What do all four of these have in common? They are characterized by a distinctive kind of personal relationship—doctor-patient, lawyer-client, teacher-student, priest-penitent—where one member was vulnerable and in need of help, and the other member promised (explicitly or implicitly) to provide just such help through healing, legal counsel, teaching, or spiritual care. Because of the imbalance of power in these relationships, great harm could come to a person if one of these professionals abused their privilege. For these fiduciary relationships to be possible, individuals and society needed to trust these professionals—to maintain confidence in their training, their competency, and most of all, their upright motives and intentions.

One of the chief means of convincing society that these professionals were trustworthy was the tradition of a public ritual, where initiates made a solemn and binding public promise prior to engaging in their work. According to the original meaning, they were *professionals* precisely because they *professed* a public oath when they commenced their career. In the case of physicians, this was, of course, the Hippocratic Oath, whereby doctors promised to use their learning, their privileges, and their powers always and only to heal the patient. Physicians solemnly swore to avoid harming the patient, to maintain confidentiality, and to avoid exploiting the patient or abusing their power, and so forth.

Following Dr. Pellegrino's speech, we stood and professed a modified version of the Hippocratic Oath—which, I regret to inform you, lacked some of the pithy language and concrete provisions of the original. With the original oath, Hippocrates founded medicine as a profession devoted entirely and exclusively to healing, explicitly excluding the deliberate injuring of patients.[4] The Hippocratic Oath implicitly suggests that iatrogenic harm—disease caused deliberately or inadvertently by medicine itself—constitutes the foundational problem in medicine and clinical ethics, a theme I will return to later on in this book.

The original oath specifically forbids the infliction of specific kinds of wounds that constitute perennial temptations for medicine. It prohibits killing (abortion and euthanasia—the paradigmatic instances of wounding), sexual exploitation, and violating patient confidentiality. By contrast, modern versions of the Hippocratic Oath—including the version administered by my medical school—discard some or all these prohibitions in favor of vague, unspecified humanitarian aspirations. For example, the oath taken by students at the University of California, Irvine, where I taught for sixteen years, was written by the students themselves—hardly an example of joining a tradition, which comes from the root *tradere*, which means "to hand on." Diverse pledges of dubious origins have today replaced a common medical creed.

We seem to want medicine to remain a profession, since the doctor is not merely a technician nor even just a humanitarian, but we don't agree on what the doctor should profess, hence the varied array of pledges. That we no longer have a common oath suggests that we no longer have a shared understanding of what it means to be a physician. Perhaps the specific oath taken should later be posted on the doctor's office wall, so future patients can at least know what their physician did or did not promise. Some patients, armed with this information, might choose to seek out a traditional Hippocratic physician, while others may be content with a technician of medical power. In any case, recent deviations from the ancient Hippocratic tradition have not, in my view, been a salutary development for the profession of medicine.

Healers can and sometimes necessarily do wound—indeed, we often heal precisely by wounding, as when a surgeon wields a scalpel. This inescapable fact rightly troubles us. We also injure through error, and we injure by means of role-confusion, like when we use our medical knowledge and skills—unethically and in violation of the oath—to participate in capital punishment or torture. Hippocrates composed his oath precisely to forestall this role confusion and to make clear to potential patients exactly how Hippocratic physicians would and would not use their knowledge and skills. We should always avoid deliberately injuring. And deliberately inflicted death is the ultimate injury, as philosopher and medical ethicist T. A. Cavanaugh explains: "The sick labor under a burden; medicine attempts to alleviate that burden. To undo the subject by killing him does not lift the burden. Rather, to do so is to take the side of illness against the patient by unwinding him. The death-dealer does disease's last work."[5]

That physicians inevitably wound makes medicine dangerous and makes a public promise—a solemn and binding oath—necessary at the outset. The central ethical norm that grounds medical practice is found in a pithy aphorism in the first chapter of Hippocrates's work *Epidemics*: "As to diseases, practice two: help or do no harm."[6] Medicine is grounded in limits, in the ability of physicians to say no to certain requests. We neglect this at our peril.

This was the long and venerable tradition I stepped into, even with only dim awareness of its full implications, that day at Georgetown's White Coat Ceremony. After professing the (modernized) oath, one by one, we walked to the stage, where a faculty member robed us in our white coat, signifying our initiation into the medical profession. A gesture that could have easily appeared forced, awkward, or stilted was carried out here with gravitas and style. Dr. Pellegrino himself put the white coat on me. Since that day, I've tried to wear it well.

Eighteen years later, I would give the White Coat Ceremony lecture to incoming students at UCI, where I was a professor in the school of medicine. My remarks echoed many of the themes I had learned from Dr. Pellegrino when I embarked on my training. I encouraged the students to focus their attention on patients and seek the internal rewards of medicine rather than external plaudits:

> From now until you retire, do not stop cultivating and reviewing your medical knowledge. We make progress through a continual critique of what we have learned. At the same time, keep in mind that knowledge alone is not enough. It's not science, but love and devotion, that transforms the world. You will alleviate pain and distress not only with a well-chosen

prescription, but also with a word of encouragement and compassion. Cultivate and maintain a breadth of interests, even while in medical school. All of your human passions and pursuits can be relevant to your professional work. After all, physicians are not robots who treat diseases; we are people who treat other people. In your clinical practice, attend with particular devotion to the abandoned patient, the lonely patient, the patient who suffers not only physical deprivations but human deprivations as well. In your work, always, always follow the light of your conscience, even when your decisions are unpopular. Guard against professional envy. Instead, focus your energies on serving your patients and assisting your colleagues. This will be success enough.

I concluded my lecture with some remarks about the unique calling of physicians:

Be absolutely convinced that you are here for a great and noble purpose. Not one of you landed here by accident. Being a physician is a way of life, not just a livelihood. Medicine is a *vocation*; it's not just a *career*. What is the difference, you might ask? Here's the best that I can explain it. Four years from now, when the dean hands you your medical degree, consider this: You are a physician not because you went to medical school; rather, you went to medical school because you are a physician.[7]

After the ceremony at Georgetown where I received my own white coat, we made our way into the courtyard for *hors d'oeuvres* and champagne. It would be some time before our school would treat us again to bubbly drinks and chocolate-covered strawberries, and we all sensed it. This was the calm before the storm. The tough realities of lectures, libraries, and labs were about to set in. Not to mention cadavers.

My first year of medical school consisted essentially of learning about the healthy human body (gross, microscopic, and neuroanatomy), biochemistry, embryology, genetics, and so on. There were a few "humanist" courses, such as "Introduction to the Patient," and "Religious Traditions in Healthcare," but the brunt of the work was in the basic sciences. The second year focused on learning about the sick human body and how to treat it: pathology (the diseases), microbiology (the bugs that attack the body), pharmacology (the drugs that eradicate the bugs and ameliorate the diseases), and so on. During these first two years, most of our time was spent studying for exams and working in labs. The final two years consisted of actual clinical training—that is, treating patients in the hospitals and clinics. These clinical years, about which I will say much more in subsequent chapters, were a trial by fire, a jump-in-and-swim apprenticeship.

In a failed attempt to convince us that ruthless competition for grades was not the norm in medical school, Georgetown had a "pass/fail" grading system. Or so they told us. "P equals MD" was the mantra, always on the tip of our tongue. When a friend appeared stressed out over next week's final, we would remind him of this truism. "Do you know your doctor's med school GPA? Or even what med school she attended? Do you care what she scored on her embryology exam?" The thinking behind the pass/fail system ran as follows: We were supposed to learn the material for its own sake and the sake of our future patients; we were all smart enough, or we would not have been admitted to medical school; since we had come this far as students, we were beyond the point of needing the prodding of grades to motivate us, and so forth. All this was true, to an extent. What we quickly realized was that this pass/fail system also included "honors," "high pass," and "low pass." Not two grades, but five. This was eerily reminiscent of our earlier academic evaluations: A, B, C, D, and F. Grades had not changed much after all.

The deans also neglected to mention that each member of the class was ranked according to academic performance—a number recorded on our transcripts to be included in residency applications. This ranking was also used to award the coveted Alpha Omega Alpha designation. "AOA," the medical student honor society, is typically required for acceptance to the most competitive residency programs. Those who consciously aim this high in medical school are known as "Gunners." Not only were Georgetown's Gunners born at the far end of the IQ bell curve, but they also possessed the motivation and drive to match their rare intellect. A few yahoos in my class wore custom-made T-shirts with "GUNNER" emblazoned on the front (picture John Belushi's "COLLEGE" sweatshirt in *Animal House*), but everyone knew these guys were not the genuine article. The real Gunners did not advertise. But they were among us. If their classmates did not figure them out, they were exposed at the pre-graduation awards ceremony a few years later as they made multiple trips across the stage to receive accolades from the various departments. Every medical school class has them: Top Guns, the best of the best.

We were told that competition at Georgetown was less ruthless than some medical schools. The atmosphere was more or less collegial; students generally helped each other out, studied together, and were little interested in seeing our classmates go down in flames. We heard stories about other schools that chilled our kind and considerate hearts: students checking out or hiding all the copies of library books needed to study for the upcoming exam; students stealing others' notebooks, binders, disks and drives; students cheating, lying, and conniving. As the rumor mill churned, we came to believe there existed medical schools where deceit, envy, conspiracy, pillage, murder, suicide, ruin, and misery were the norm. For example, gross anatomy lab exams typically consist of questions about anatomic structures identified with small pins placed in the cadavers' corresponding body part. Reports circulated of a notorious practice perpetrated by malicious students who surreptitiously moved these pins to other structures as they progressed through the exam, thus dooming every student behind them to confusion. I was glad this sort of thing did not happen at my medical school.

My first patient was already dead. My only job involved painstakingly dissecting her lifeless corpse in the anatomy lab, reducing every inch of her body to tatters until there was nothing left to cut. I took her apart; I pulled her to pieces; but I never learned her name. And she never knew mine.

As far as I knew, she was an anonymous person with no social or psychological life, no family, no community, no context. Merely a lifeless body lying on a steel table. Unfortunately, medical students observe death before we observe life. I only later learned in the surgical operating room that a living body looks very little like a dead one. There is a strange historical myth, perpetuated still today, that early men of science in the late-eighteenth and early-nineteenth centuries pioneered dissection of cadavers by stealing bodies from graves to get around religious or legal prohibitions of the practice. It's a myth because, while some scientific pioneers did rob graves for this purpose, it was entirely unnecessary. The practice of human dissection was neither legally prohibited nor frowned upon by the Church and civil authorities at the time.

Dissection had been forbidden earlier in ancient Greece and Rome, and likewise prohibited in Islamic societies. It was the medieval Scholastics who first permitted the practice under the theological justification that the soul, not the body, was unique to humans. Resistance to pathological anatomy in the early days of modern science came neither from the Church nor the law nor society.[8] Ironically, resistance to dissection in those days came from medicine itself.[9] Dissecting clinics existed in hospitals in Vienna, Pavia, and Paris from the 1750s, but these were held in suspicion by the birth of new medical clinics.

Strange to say, there was no need for anatomists to rob graves, and yet they did. Why? The grave-robbing doctors of the early nineteenth century wanted to see themselves as seeking a prohibited knowledge and exposing the inadequacy of the old ways of thinking for the new society,[10] as bioethicist Jeffrey Bishop explains in his book *The Anticipatory Corpse*: "The dead body became the fetish of medicine; the desired object was knowledge, and the dead body came to stand for that knowledge."[11] Pioneers of modern anatomy cultivated a self-conception that science and medicine needed to venture into unseen realms to acquire secret—even "forbidden"—knowledge by penetrating deep within the previously inviolable space of the body. The philosopher Michel Foucault describes the false historical tale that was spun to sustain this self-understanding of medicine:

> For a hundred and fifty years, the same explanation had been repeated: medicine could gain access to that which founded it scientifically only by circumventing, slowly and prudently, one major obstacle, the opposition of religion, morality, and stubborn prejudice to the opening up of corpses. Pathological anatomy had had not more than a shadowy existence, on the edge of prohibition, sustained only by that courage in the face of malediction peculiar to seekers after secret knowledge; dissection was carried out only under cover of the shadowy twilight, in great fear of the dead. . . . A fine transmutation of the corpse had taken place: gloomy respect had condemned it to putrefaction, to the dark work of destruction; in the boldness of the gesture that violated only to reveal, to bring to the light of day, the corpse became the brightest moment in the figures of truth. Knowledge spins where once larva was formed.[12]

Never mind that the early anatomists had no difficulty in the middle of the eighteenth century in carrying out autopsies, as Foucault goes on to explain in his classic study *The Birth of the Clinic*: "There was no shortage of corpses in the eighteenth century, no need to rob graves or to perform anatomical black masses; one was already in the full light of dissection."[13] Nevertheless, the early anatomists felt the need to convince themselves and others that they were doing something forbidden to usher in this new science of the human body. Apparently, secret knowledge equated to special knowledge, available only to the few scientists daring enough to violate ancient taboos.

The practice of dissecting a dead body remains today a rite of passage for fresh medical students. The first thing I noticed when I walked into the lab was the smell of formaldehyde, which permeated everything (and everyone) that entered the room. No amount of washing could adequately rid our clothes of that smell. Even after two showers, my wife could smell it on my hair. The second thing I noticed was, of course, the body bags on the tables.

With due deference to ancient societies that looked askance at human dissection, I would question the moral sensibility of anyone who did not at least pause to wonder whether dissecting a dead body might be an irreverent act, perhaps one that should not be allowed. Respect for our mortal remains has been a permanent feature of human history from the beginning. The specific means of disposing of dead bodies differ across various cultures, but all share an innate sense that some ritual act of regard is necessary here. The human body can be desecrated in death, just as it can in life.

The penultimate lines of Homer's *Iliad* describe how the indomitable Achilles drags the brave Hector's dead body through the streets of Troy. Line after line of wanton death and destruction in the Trojan War, described in gruesome detail by the ancient bard, ends with this ultimate act of disrespect for the human body. The reader senses that amidst all the carnage of this poem, this is somehow the most brutal moment. Even more than the fear of death itself, Homer's war heroes feared having their dead body left on the battlefield as food for the dogs. In the poignant final scene, Hector's royal father, Priam, grasps the hand of the man who killed his son and desperately begs Achilles to return Hector's body for a proper burial.

Consider this: Achilles did far less physical damage to Hector's body than I did to another woman's body in gross anatomy lab. We dissected her with painstaking detail: Each structure was subjected to the knife. By the end, very little of her remains actually remained intact. Every bit of tissue had been opened, disconnected, removed, spliced. If this was not desecration, what is?

And yet, there is a difference between Achilles's act and that of a medical student performing a dissection. Gross anatomy lab is often defended on the instrumental grounds that it produces a great good: essential knowledge for future physicians. It thus contributes to the lives of future patients who will rely on our knowledge. This is true, but such utilitarian reasoning is not enough. The two acts differ in their total meaning, in the attitude and approach to the dead body. Achilles intended to destroy; the medical student intends to discover.

The students I discussed this with were, without exception, profoundly grateful to the person who donated his or her body for this purpose. We approached the dead bodies—at least initially—with wonder and awe. Georgetown has a tradition of offering a Catholic Mass every year for the repose of the souls of deceased donors and for their families, who invariably express appreciation for this gesture.

The human body is an astonishing work of art—arguably the most beautiful thing in the natural world. The wisdom of the body, which I began to really understand only by dissecting it, consisted of a million secrets, none of which was divulged readily. Any gain in anatomic knowledge required probing, coaxing, and teasing it out with scalpel and scissors. I learned less in a week of studying anatomy books than in an hour of cadaver dissection. Pictures and diagrams are no replacement for the real thing, turned over between your fingers.

Gross anatomy lab totally absorbed my mind. At home, after a long day of many hours in gross lab, I would try to think about something other than medical school for a while, only to find myself staring at my forearm at the dinner table, flexing one finger at a time, watching tendon and muscle move underneath the skin. "Are you studying your arm *again*?" my wife would interrupt.

Snapping out of my trance, I would sheepishly reply, "Sorry . . . can't help it."

"You're obsessed."
"Yep."

"There are no locker rooms. Where are we supposed to change for gross lab?"

"Most students opt to change next to the lockers in the hall. Or if you're not comfortable with this, you can use the bathrooms."

The case for changing in the hall included the claim that it was a "bonding experience" among classmates. Failing to understand how this would further my professional solidarity with my female classmates, I made my way to the small men's room, where a dozen other guys had crammed themselves. After donning the clothes that would be sacrificed to formaldehyde, I made my way back through the hall past the bonding bras and briefs on either side.

The first day, the atmosphere was somber. A feeling of quiet trepidation pervaded the room as we thought of what we were about to do. We uncovered the chest first. It appeared as the off-human color of life drained away: neither gray nor brown, but somewhere in between, a washed out yellow-beige. Putting scalpel to skin, we began to cut. The knife drew no blood, for no blood could flow from a corpse. Our pace gradually quickened as we went to work dissecting. In the days that followed, the atmosphere relaxed: The volume rose, laughter returned.

A few months later, the days of gross anatomy were winding down. Each group of four students was ready to be through with our cadaver, to finish the last section of the course: head and neck anatomy. One day near the end of the course, we uncovered the face, until then hidden under a plastic bag. The somber atmosphere of day one suddenly returned. It took us off guard. Had we gradually disregarded what we knew at the beginning? Had we forgotten what we had been doing for the past three months? "Man grows used to everything, the scoundrel," said Fyodor Dostoevsky's Raskolnikov in *Crime and*

Punishment.[14] How quickly we had accustomed ourselves to dissecting the dead.

Before we cut again, we looked at the face, that mysterious place from which the human personality radiates most fully. We looked at the mouth that had smiled and the eyes that had cried, now dry and drained and stiff. This face—the seat of the senses and the window into the soul—arrested us for a few moments. The eyes gave us pause. Then, as instructed, after a few moments we picked up our scalpels and applied them to the face.

It is strange, the things you find when you carve open dead bodies. One man's liver was rock hard, cirrhotic, probably from years of alcohol abuse. We discovered tumors, remnants of old surgeries, food still in the stomach, stool still in the colon, a spleen six times the normal size. One of the brains, not having been adequately preserved with sufficient formaldehyde, had begun to liquefy. After removing the top of the skull like a hat, we watched, disgusted, as the brain slid partially out, oozing in a semi-liquid sludge toward the floor. Eating lunch was sometimes difficult after anatomy lab.

The day we dissected the genitals—not an easy endeavor, mind you—we discovered that one cadaver had a prosthesis inside his penis. Until then, I was naïvely unaware that such devices existed. They are among the remedies for men with erectile dysfunction (in common parlance, impotence), and they come in various and sundry models: some inflate and deflate, while others remain permanently erect. (The latter type folds down when not in use, in case you were wondering.) One of our professors, a urologist, was delighted with this find. Students gathered around him as he held up the device, turned it over in the light, all the while explaining to us the year, make, and model. One could see a gleam in his eye as he admired the materials and craftsmanship. Urologists, I thought, must be a unique breed.

The early formative experience of human cadaver dissection powerfully shapes—for good or ill—the ethos and imagination of physicians. It sets the tone for the entire practice of modern medicine.

Beginning with gross anatomy lab, the dead body becomes medicine's template for understanding the living organism. The medical student constructs his knowledge of the human body on the foundation of the static, frozen-in-time, lifeless, decontextualized corpse. This "dead" knowledge is later overlayed onto the dynamic bodies of the living. The corpse serves as the normative starting point against which the dynamic flux of life is understood.

But this gets things backwards. Consequently, the living body comes to be seen as a machine—as dead matter somehow kept in motion by mysterious forces we do not understand. Consider, for example, this dubious claim from a contemporary textbook of medical physiology: "The human being is actually an automaton, and the fact that we are sensing, feeling, and knowledgeable beings is part of this automatic sequence of life."[15] This reductionist view of the living body as mere dead mechanism is not new: We find the roots of this cramped attitude in the advent of modern medical science, including physiology, which is supposed to study the dynamic processes of life. The dead/mechanistic model ails medicine to this day.

Claude Bernard (1813–1878) was the most preeminent physiologist of the nineteenth century and pioneered the concept of homeostasis, among other important discoveries. In his classic work *An Introduction to the Study of Experimental Medicine*, Bernard argued that the living body must be understood by studying the mechanisms of death—even by inducing death. For Bernard, there is no fundamental difference between inorganic and organic matter: Both obey the same deterministic laws of physics and chemistry. He therefore referred to the living human body as an "animal machine," much as today's physiology textbook refers to it as an "automaton."

Bernard claimed that we cannot know *why* bodies work—science tells us nothing about purpose—but only *how* they work; we know only the means but not the ends of human life. This knowledge provides not wisdom about life but power over nature. As he put it, "We know absolutely nothing of the essence even of life; but we shall nevertheless regulate vital phenomena as soon as we know enough of their necessary conditions."[16] In short, while we cannot comprehend life, we can nevertheless learn to control it.

To gain such knowledge, Bernard was a proponent of vivisection—the dissection of living animals (before the advent of anesthesia)—to advance the science of physiology. He once killed the family dog by vivisection which, as you might imagine, did not much please his wife and daughters. His wife later separated from him and campaigned against vivisection. Bernard's argument for this gruesome practice is striking, indeed disturbing, coming from such an eminent figure in the history of medical science:

> We have succeeded in discovering the laws of inorganic matter only by penetrating into inanimate bodies and machines; similarly we shall succeed in learning the laws of properties of living matter only by displacing living organs in order to get into their inner environment. After dissecting cadavers, then, we must necessarily dissect living beings, to uncover the inner or hidden parts of the organisms and see them work; to this sort of operation we give the name vivisection, and without this mode of investigation, neither physiology nor scientific medicine is possible; to learn how man and animals live, we cannot avoid seeing great numbers of them die, because the mechanisms of life can be unveiled and proved only by knowledge of the mechanisms of death.[17]

This comes straight from the pen of the founding father of physiology, the study of living organisms: Death is necessary for the advance of medicine. Against his detractors, Bernard argued that just as "prejudices clinging to respect for corpses long halted the progress of anatomy," in the same way vivisection encounters prejudiced detractors. However, such people merely "deny experimental medicine, i.e., scientific medicine" and therefore their arguments unworthy of a response.[18] Raise moral objections to killing animals (or humans) to advance the study of life, and you will be classed among the backward—an anti-science rube standing athwart medical progress.

Bernard stopped just short of advocating human vivisection, including of criminals, though he did argue for experimentation on human beings immediately after capital punishment by decapitation. Men of science cannot afford the luxury of squeamishness, after all. In his words, "A physiologist is not a man of fashion, he is a man of science, absorbed by the scientific idea which he pursues: he no longer hears the cry of animals, he no longer sees the blood that flows, he sees only his idea and perceives only organisms concealing problems which he intends to solve."[19] To study life, the scientist must suppress human feelings and moral reservations. But do we really want physicians who are well-practiced in this?

While modern medical training did not, for the most part, follow Bernard into the morally dubious realms of vivisection, we did adopt his mechanistic philosophy that views the living body as no more than passive matter-in-motion—a machine that is not fundamentally different in life than in death. The physician is trained to view the human body primarily in terms of dead dissected parts that can subsequently be reconstructed, rather than as a self-directed, coordinated, dynamic, living whole greater than the sum of its parts. But as psychiatrist, philosopher, and neuroscientist Iain McGilchrist argues in his magisterial two-volume work, *The Matter with Things*, the mechanistic view of biology espoused by Bernard and his intellectual descendants is untenable, given what we have learned about living organisms from experiment and observation:

> I would suggest that there are broadly six features that stand out in the language inevitably used by biologists, rather than by physicists or chemists, time and time again, year after year, decade after decade, century after century . . . language used to describe what they actually see, but which stands in blatant

contradiction to the metaphor of the machine. What are they? References to (1) *actively co-ordinated processes*, expressing a sense of (2) *wholeness*, inextricably linked with (3) *values*, (4) *meaning* and (5) *purpose*—each leading separately and together, to the phenomenon of (6) *self-realisation*. None of these get to be applied to my car.[20] [emphasis in original]

In a machine, the parts are constructed to make up the whole. But in an organism, the whole constructs and reconstructs the parts. Examples from human biology could be multiplied indefinitely, but to illustrate, I'll mention just one fascinating aspect of fetal development. The following shows how dynamic form and function are prior to static structure in biology. The heart has a left and right side separated by a wall called a septum. The right side of the heart receives blood from the body and sends it to the lungs for oxygenation, while the left side receives oxygenated blood from the lungs and sends it back out to the rest of the body. Blood flows in opposite directions through the left and right sides. Before the wall between the left and right side of the heart even develops in the fetus, blood is already flowing in two distinct but opposite currents through the primitive heart. This dynamic flow creates the framework for the development of the septum (or wall), as biologist Craig Holdrege explains:

> The blood flowing through the right and left sides of the heart do not mix, but stream and loop by each other, just as two currents in a body of water. In the "still water zone" between the two currents, the septum dividing the two chambers forms. Thus the movement of the blood gives the parameters for the inner differentiation of the heart, just as the looping heart redirects the flow of blood.[21]

The heart's dynamic flow precedes and directs the construction of its static structure, as is fitting for a living organism rather than a dead machine: Human life is a process before it is a thing. Unlike the parts of a machine, "the liver, the heart, the kidneys are not assembled, but come into ever more defined being as the whole living organism grows," as McGilchrist explains. Furthermore, "the relationship between the parts don't go to *make up* the whole, but *derive from* the existence of the whole"[22] (emphasis in original).

In other words, biological life is an intricately choreographed dance that cannot be captured in a photograph. Trying to get at its essence by dissecting it into ever smaller parts and examining each part in isolation, as we would do with a machine, "would be like trying to account of the unique quality, the power, and yes, the *life* of a piece of music by examining each note, or at most a phrase, in ever greater detail, outside the flow of the whole work, in the hope that by this 'drilling down', as we say, there at last we will find the secret"[23] (emphasis in original). The machine model of the human body persists in our imagination not because it is true, but because "it encourages the sense that we can easily understand what life is and learn to control it"[24]—a tempting proposition for our Faustian age. But because the mechanistic view of the body as a dead machine built up of distinct parts is not true to life, the cadaveric starting point is not necessarily the only—much less the best—approach to medical education. But it is the one we have deliberately chosen, and we now reap the fruits.

The other feature of the first two years that deserves mention is somewhat less glamorous. Memorization. There is no way around it. As rigorous and challenging as my undergraduate years at the University of Notre Dame had been, the demands of studying during the first year of medical school caught me by surprise. I was not prepared for the minutiae, the innumerable details, the sheer volume of information that I was expected to master.

My method involved a whiteboard—my secret weapon. I would first fill the whiteboard with diagrams, charts, and lists, then stare at it, read it, close my eyes, and pace the room muttering to myself, trying to cram its contents into my memory. Then, out came the eraser, followed by more repetitive murmuring, and an attempt to reproduce on the whiteboard the information I had just erased. This went on for hours on end. I rarely enjoyed it; often, I despised it. But I told myself, an adequate fund of knowledge is indispensable for a physician, and the exams were far from easy. "Can you believe they expected us to remember *that*?" was a common post-exam complaint.

It was not that the material itself was overly difficult to comprehend. It was simply that there was so much material. By the middle of second year—the doldrums, when hospitals and patients seemed worlds away—I had asked myself countless times the question: What have I gotten myself into? Why on earth am I doing this?

After asking this for the thousandth time, I would take another swig of coffee, rub my eyes, pick up my pen, and return to my whiteboard. I have come this far . . . I have invested so much . . . I might as well finish. So I reasoned. And pressed on. But there were days when I didn't know why.

We were fed small morsels of clinical experience during the first two years. These tastes of what was to come—a little contact with patients, some time in a clinic or hospital—whet our appetite for third-year clinical rotations. They kept us motivated as we slogged on through thick textbooks and reams of lecture notes.

During my second year, in my first real experience in a hospital, I saw a man knock on death's door. Enthralled, I watched a cardiologist calmly and deftly bring him back from the precipice. The incident began while a classmate and I were enjoying a slow day in Dr. Zamanzi's clinic. The class was Physical Diagnosis, where second-year students learn the art of examining patients and taking a thorough medical history. Our instructor had invited the two of us to his clinic, where he demonstrated diagnostic techniques on his patients, then let us listen to the heart, shine lights in the eyes, peer into the ears, and so on. Zamanzi's pager went off, and he disappeared from the room for a few minutes, leaving the two of us rookies sitting awkwardly alone with a patient. The Real Doctor returned a few moments later and motioned us out of the room. This patient's appointment would have to wait.

"Come with me to the hospital. One of my patients just coded." We had only a vague notion of what this meant, or what was to come next. Hospitals have various "codes" that are classified by a color indicating the nature of the problem, all of them emergencies. In this case, the code blue was a cardiac arrest due to an abnormal heart rhythm. In our fourth year, we would ourselves learn how to "run the code."

The hospital was conveniently located next door to Dr. Zamanzi's office. We strode over in haste. When we arrived, the patient's room was already a hubbub of activity. The other medical student and I made our way to the corner, trying to stay out of the way. There we remained for the next forty minutes, a couple of useless flies on the wall.

On the bed lay a massive naked and unconscious man who was forty-four years old and dying. From his mouth, a breathing tube was attached to an inflatable oval ball, which a nurse was squeezing steadily at a rate of twenty per minute, "bagging" the patient. His chest rose with each compression, the nurse's hands breathing for the patient. Another nurse held a defibrillator paddle in each hand—those mysterious magic wands of modern medicine. Familiar to the lay public from television and the movies, these are often believed to somehow "jumpstart" the heart, usually after many attempts and just when the audience is about to give up hope.

Dr. Zamanzi took over for the other hospital physician and began directing traffic with strong, sure-fire commands. And there was a lot of traffic to direct: I counted thirteen healthcare personnel in the one-bed hospital room, not including the medical students. Each person had a task: bagging, shocking, compressing the chest to pump blood, giving IV medications, checking the pulse with a small handheld Doppler device. One person's job was simply to write down everything Dr. Zamanzi said, verify that each order was carried out, and record the time intervals between medication doses. Everyone in the room watched the monitors intently for any change in the patient's "vital signs"—heart rate, respirations, blood pressure—signs which, without chest compressions and bagging, were nonexistent. The EKG monitor showed the characteristic irregular jagged pattern of ventricular fibrillation, a disorganized cardiac rhythm where the heart beats far too quickly to fill adequately with blood, and far too chaotically to propel blood into circulation. But even this frightfully crazed rhythm is better than no rhythm. This was "shockable": The patient's heart was "fibrillating," but the magic paddles were part of a modern electrically powered medical wonder, the "defibrillator."

By contrast, it is useless to shock a flatline, a heart with no rhythmic activity—contrary to what you see on television. Also contrary to popular belief, the defibrillator does not "jumpstart" a non-beating heart. Paradoxically, it actually stops the heart's activity altogether. For a brief moment after shocking, one sees the flatline where before there was rapid activity. The hope is that by passing a massive current of electricity through the chest, one can reset the heart's own electrical conduction system. It's a bit like hitting restart on your computer when the software is jammed up. After the momentary flatline, one waits eagerly for a "normal sinus rhythm" to appear—the apple of a cardiologist's well-trained eye. But in this patient, despite shock after dramatic shock, the jagged chaos continued.

"Stand clear, clear . . . I'm shocking, shocking!" the nurse with the paddles would announce. The bagger, IV-pusher, and pulse-searcher would stand away, as the shocker depressed the buttons on the paddles, sending 360 joules of current through the patient's barrel chest.

His enormous body convulsed. All three hundred pounds of flesh seemed to rise off the bed with each wave of electricity.

"Still no pulse."

"Give another hundred and fifty milligrams of Amiodarone," Dr. Zamanzi ordered. "How long since the last Epi dose?"

"Four minutes," the recording nurse with the clipboard replied.

"Give another dose of Epinephrine."

"One milligram Epinephrine," announced the IV pusher, as he depressed the syringe.

"Still no pulse."

"Okay, let's go again," Zamanzi would say. He seemed never to lose confidence.

"Stand clear, clear . . . I'm shocking, shocking . . ."

This cycle went on and on.

Amazed at the cool efficiency of it all, at the relentless perseverance of the team in the face of continued failure to resuscitate, I stood in awe. After several rounds of this, I began to wonder whether it would work. Perhaps it would not happen here in the real world the way it happened on television. I wondered whether this might turn out to be a hopeless exercise, a dogged refusal to accept the inevitable. This thought was not entirely without merit: The question of precisely when to discontinue a code, I later learned, cannot be answered with any certainty. When the line goes flat, eventually, the doctor must throw in the towel. There are few hard and fast conventions; how long the physician continues before he declares the patient dead is largely up to him.

But this was not to be this patient's fate. At least, not that day. Eventually his pulse returned, faint, the rhythm not quite normal, but regular enough to pump blood to his oxygen-starved tissues. As the patient stabilized, the intense cadenced activity in the room—shock, drug, check, shock—gradually slackened, and the code team progressively dispersed. Dr. Zamanzi stepped out to talk with the patient's family. He returned with a look of frustrated exhaustion. Surprised, given that he had just saved someone's life in such grand heroic fashion, I wondered why he looked so haggard.

"I didn't think he'd make it," I told him.

"I knew he would," the doctor replied. "But the family wants to know why I haven't cured him. This is a patient with cardiomyopathy and congestive heart failure. That was the fourth time he's arrested this year. He will not change his diet, exercise, or even take his medications. His family insists that I 'fix' him. It's absurd. This man refuses to help himself. I've explained to them over and over that he is going to die. They will not accept it." He sighed. "There is nothing more I can do for him. He is going to die soon."

This cardiac code fits the popular image of modern medicine. Armed with expert scientific knowledge, with the arsenal of high technology at his disposal, the good physician battles the evil enemies—disease and death—in a dramatic struggle to "save" the patient, who is usually a passive victim. Illness is largely something that "happens" to someone, and it is the doctor's job to fight it, to vanquish the disease with weapons of technological wizardry and infallible know-how.

This understanding of medicine, I came to realize, is mostly wrong. I began to comprehend this as my medical training progressed, as I saw more and more patients who brought misery upon themselves. To say this is neither to "blame the victim" nor to argue that all disease is the result of a lazy, hedonistic, or irrational lifestyle. Rather, it is simply to acknowledge that each of us bears no small responsibility for our own health. This concept lies at the very root of Western medicine; it is central to the philosophy of the father of medicine, Hippocrates himself.

Hippocrates understood a basic truth that many in medicine have forgotten: The patient is the primary healer; the physician occupies merely a supporting role. Although we are reluctant to admit this, our health is, to a significant extent, our own responsibility. Many want to live, eat, drink, and do as they wish; when they suffer the natural consequences, they look to someone else to cure them. But modern medicine, despite its undeniable achievements, offers very few real cures. More often than not, the physician manages a patient's disease, mitigates symptoms, and minimizes complications. Only rarely do we cure.

This is why Hippocrates always began treatment with an individualized "regimen" of diet, physical activity, rest and reprieve in the proper environment, and so on. Only then did he look to drugs or surgery. Granted, he had fewer medical or surgical options to employ than we do today. His method, however, has much to recommend it. During medical school, I was taught a great deal about fighting disease but almost nothing about promoting health. The gold-standard textbook, *Harrison's Principles of Internal Medicine*, does not even have the word "health" in the index; the book is basically a voluminous compendium of disease. In my opinion, people's dissatisfaction with mainstream medicine's focus on fighting disease rather than promoting health partially explains the ongoing interest in alternative and complementary medicine.

I began to see some of modern medicine's shortcomings when I witnessed this case. Here was a relatively young patient who received all the benefits that medical technology had to offer. Yet a few months later, he was dead. The victory I witnessed that day was only a brief delay before the final defeat. Ultimately, this patient lost because he refused to help himself.

The failures of medicine often become clearest, ironically, at its moments of greatest triumph.

CHAPTER 3

See One, Do One, Teach One

They certainly give very strange and newfangled names to diseases.

—Plato[1]

Although there was some flirtation here and there, medicine did not really seduce me during the pre-clinical years. My courtship really began during the third year, when I was introduced to my new love in her own home—the modern hospital. But before I courted her, I had to learn her language.

It is no secret that physicians speak a different language than the rest of mankind. Learning it is a baffling experience. Some have suggested, not without reason, that medical jargon's very purpose is to mystify patients and elevate the physician as the possessor of impossibly technical knowledge the lay public cannot comprehend. In Molière's satirical play *The Imaginary Invalid* (1673), the pompous doctor responds to the question of why opium induces sleep with the tautological, pseudo-learned Latinate "explanation" that it has a *virtus dormitiva*: "Because there is in it a dormitive virtue, whose nature is to lull the senses."[2] Oh, okay.

To master the foreign language, it is not enough to diligently study a medical dictionary (although this was the most useful book that I purchased my first year), since much of the language is not found there. The medical dictionary will serve you well during the pre-clinical years, but once you are in the hospital, the language changes again. Acronyms replace phrases, abbreviations replace proper terminology, trade names replace generic ones for drugs, and, of course, slang makes its way into the lexicon. There are no dictionaries for the acronyms, abbreviations, or slang.

The experience is analogous to learning a foreign language in college. One can dedicate a few years to studying nothing but intensive Spanish and become fairly proficient. But when the student of college Spanish takes this knowledge to Spain or Mexico, he quickly learns that his method of speaking sounds significantly different from the natives. He may have mastered the formal aspects of grammar; he may have a respectable vocabulary and know all the proper verb conjugations. But his language sounds, to the native speaker, slow and stilted and somewhat artificial. It is not merely that he has an "accent" and lacks the precise pronunciation of the native speaker. Rather, it is that the natives do not follow the rules of grammar to a T: They use contractions, abbreviations, slang, and figures of speech. The same phenomenon happens in medical school. This is why when I arrived at the hospital in the beginning of the third year, I felt like a foreigner, and often like a fool. Patients have a similar experience around doctors who chronically fail to drop the medical jargon at the bedside, where it serves to mystify instead of clarify.

I knew the names of the diseases, the drugs, the anatomy, and all the rest. After all, I had literally added thousands upon thousands of new words to my vocabulary in the past two years. Yet it was immediately clear that I still did not sound like the residents and attendings—like the native speakers. "Nobody calls it furosemide; it's Lasix," a kindly resident informed me. A-gram, not arteriogram. MI, not myocardial infarct . . .

As if the language was not confusing enough, as a third-year student, I had to learn the fine art of navigating the hospital hierarchy. Apart from the military, the most rigid and complicated hierarchies in the United States are found in teaching hospitals. On balance, this is not entirely bad. For many reasons, things must be this way if patients are to get proper care, if responsibilities are to be appropriately delegated, and if new physicians are to be suitably trained. There must be some kind of power structure, a chain of command to make this endlessly complicated institution function. Though, as everyone has experienced, bureaucratic hierarchies have their own attendant pathologies.

The difficulties for the uninitiated student come about because the hierarchical relationships are never explicitly spelled out, never explained to him; there is no orientation in cultural etiquette, no crash course in customs and taboos. Most medical students have to stumble through, paging the wrong person, asking the wrong questions, doing work that should be done by a senior, and neglecting work that was their responsibility. The quicker one picks up on the unspoken nuances, the better; but the learning curve can be painful.

The hierarchy, in brief, goes something like this. At the top are the "attendings," physicians that work in the hospital and have faculty appointments in the medical school to supervise and teach the residents and students. The department chair or division chief is the attending perched at the peak of the pyramid. Under the attendings are the heterogeneous group known as "residents," physicians who are completing the post-medical school training in their particular specialty. The residents are medical doctors, but they are not yet board-certified in a specific field; this is precisely what residency is training them for. Residency can last three to five years or more.

The resident's older cousins form an in-between layer—above ordinary residents but below attendings: These are the "fellows." A fellow is a board-certified doctor who has completed residency but is doing additional training to become certified in a sub-specialty. For example, an internal medicine doctor may go on to do a fellowship in infectious disease, or a general surgeon may continue with a fellowship in transplant surgery. A fellowship typically requires another two to four years after residency.

The first-year resident is known as the "intern"—the hospital's beast of burden. The senior resident in charge of a service is known as the "chief" resident. Interns, residents, and fellows are collectively known as the "house staff" and individually known as "house officers." They receive a modest stipend for their work, which creeps up incrementally every year. Considering the hours that house officers put in, the money usually amounts to less than the minimum wage.

Finally, at the bottom of the totem pole, are the medical students. Third-year students receive no special designation; they are just third-year students or MS3s (the older term "clerks" has fallen out of fashion). Fourth-year students spend part of the year completing "acting internships" during which they are given clinical responsibilities similar to an intern; then they are called "AIs," or at some schools, "Sub-Is." It goes without saying that medical students are not paid. Quite the contrary, they shell out large sums of money, usually resulting in considerable debt, for the privilege of working under the house staff and attendings. At Georgetown, a third-year or fourth-year medical student could often work a schedule comparable to a resident—between eighty and one hundred hours per week on many rotations.

The nuances of the hierarchy are endless. While doing a psychiatry rotation as a fourth-year, I was working with two psychiatry fellows and one third-year student. Over the past few weeks, I had developed a rather congenial relationship with the fellows, bolstered by the fact that I had chosen psychiatry as my future field. The third-year student was new on the service, and he attempted the same convivial approach that he saw the fourth-year student taking. This irritated the fellows. Apparently, his place in the hierarchy, only slightly below my own, did not allow him to engage in the same familiarity and light bantering. "He doesn't get it," one of them observed. "He's trying to act like you," he told me, "and be 'just one of the guys.' But he's only a third-year."

"Yeah. He's going to have trouble this year," the other concurred.

This hierarchical hair-splitting was still beyond my grasp. Grateful that I was at least on their good side, I wondered what other residents I had worked with said about me when I was not in the room. Had I too committed the cardinal sin of over-familiarity?

"It's difficult, you know, navigating the intricate hierarchy," I offered in the other student's defense. "When you're a third-year, no one explains any of this to you."

"Yeah, but he's been doing this for over three months now. If he doesn't figure things out soon, he'll find this year very difficult," the fellow surmised.

Just when I thought I had figured out the system, the schedule, and the routine in the foreign culture of Georgetown University Hospital, they shipped me off to a different community hospital for my next rotation. Suddenly, the charts were not in the same place, the protocol for presenting patients was different, the expectations and responsibilities were altered, and the hierarchical maze, which I was just beginning to master, was all thrown out of whack. Without fail, every four weeks, a new culture shock hit: from surgery to pediatrics, from a university to a community hospital to an HMO clinic, from the rich to the poor side of town. Without fail, everything changed on the first of the month.

"You paged an attending?" the resident asked, looking annoyed at me. "You're not supposed to do that. At this hospital, only attendings page attendings, or if need be, the chief resident."

"Sorry. We did it all the time at Georgetown."

"Things are different here."

"I see."

In medical school, when you try to be proactive, sometimes you are applauded, other times you are reprimanded. Try as you might, it is often difficult to figure out the relevant difference between the two situations. You learn to roll with the punches in this school of hard (and inconsistent) knocks. The clinical years are as much about learning to make rapid adjustments in relatively inconsequential matters as they are about learning to make medical decisions in matters of grave consequence.

The culture shock of starting the third year was not limited to the hospital's foreign language or the social hierarchy. Local habits of dress also took some time to get used to. First, there was the white coat. This deceptively simple garment is laden with symbolism. One cannot don a doctor's white coat without at once feeling different. It symbolizes scientific expertise, clinical detachment, and perhaps most of all, the physician's authority. Patients respond to the white coat often with deference, at times with fear. There is a well-documented medical phenomenon dubbed "white coat hypertension": It has often been observed that many patients consistently have higher measured blood pressures at the doctor's office than when measured at home. Studies have explained this in terms of the anxiety provoked by the physician's white coat, which causes an elevation in blood pressure at the clinic or hospital.

Donning the white coat for the first time, I felt a strange mixture of pride and confidence, combined with a feeling that there was a total disconnect between my actual clinical abilities and the symbolic message conveyed by the garment. I felt like a pretender, like an anthropologist in a foreign culture donning the tribal chieftain's headdress. I had studied the culture and understood the role of the chieftain, yet I was still a foreigner and not quite prepared for the responsibility symbolized by the white coat.

The white coat was not only heavily laden with symbolism; it was quite literally heavily laden. The average third-year medical student's white coat weighs about eight pounds. The coats are generously outfitted with large pockets for pens, penlights, stethoscopes, smartphones, reflex hammers, scissors and tape for dressing changes, and, heaviest of all, pocket reference books. Some rookie students included more esoteric paraphernalia in their pockets, such as tuning forks to test hearing and vibration sense, or ophthalmoscopes and blood pressure cuffs, just in case there were none hanging on the wall by the patient's bedside. These new tools of the trade weighed down the otherwise light white coat considerably. While wearing it, I kept feeling like I had forgotten to take off my backpack.

As time went by, we students learned to trim down our load. As our knowledge base grew, the pocketbooks were placed back upon the shelf. As our physical exam became more focused and we became more proficient with our tools, we tossed the reflex hammer out for all but our neurology rotation and learned to use the edge of our stethoscope head to test reflexes. After a while there was no more need to carry around the *Tarascon Pocket Pharmacopoeia* or *The Washington Manual of Medical Therapeutics*. Many of the senior residents limited their pocket contents to a pen and a stethoscope. The rest was in their heads. We envied their trim approach to the tools of the trade.

In stark contrast to the weighty new feel of the white coat was the naked new feel of the hospital scrubs. Wearing these ultra-functional, ultra-cool garments for the first time gave me the feeling not that I had forgotten to remove my backpack, but that I had forgotten to change out of pajamas before coming to work. (Sort of like that recurring dream of arriving at school on the first day, only to look down and realize that I was not wearing any pants.) I felt naked in scrubs and had the constant urge to check my fly, only to discover again that there was no fly to check, but merely the drawstring, without which my scrub pants could have fit another person inside. Tall and lean, I had to wear XLs to accommodate my long legs, but this size included a spare twenty inches in the waist. The drawstring was my friend.

Although I never got around to buying a pair, most students complemented their scrubs with a pair of hush puppy shoes. These thick-soled-rubber-slip-on-without-laces black shoes provided luxurious padding underneath the heels of the retractor-holding students' tired feet while we stood for hours in the operating room. The bare-bones materials combined easy washability with rapid drying. Wearing these, one could discard the blue disposable booties, since blood and guts that dripped from the operating table could easily be hosed off the hush puppies between surgeries. Those of us who settled for sneakers had no choice but to protect them from red stains by taking on and off the blue booties.

So much for local customs of dress. Like everything else in the initially foreign hospital, before long, the enculturated medical student began to feel comfortably at home wearing the strange new garments.

My third-year clerkships included three months of internal medicine, three months of surgery, six weeks of pediatrics, six weeks of obstetrics and gynecology, and a month each of family medicine, neurology, and psychiatry. My fourth-year clerkships included three required AI months: one in medicine, one in surgery, one in a field of my choice, and a required month of emergency medicine. The rest of the fourth year consisted of elective clinical rotations, for which I chose neuroradiology, medical ethics, and additional psychiatry rotations.

Each student was assigned a small number of patients, usually between three and six, whom we followed closely. We were expected to know everything medically relevant about our patients: their history, medications, results of lab tests and radiological studies, allergies, and of course, their diseases and disorders. We spent extra time reading about these diseases to be prepared to answer questions about them. As the third year progressed, we were also expected to suggest reasonable treatment plans or diagnostic tests for our patients, thus becoming more engaged not just in diagnosis but treatment.

During the clinical years, students were part of a medical "team" that usually included one or two interns, a senior resident, often another student or a fourth-year AI, and an attending who was involved to a greater or lesser degree—depending on the situation or the specialty—in the day-to-day care of the patients. The senior resident oversaw all patients on the service and typically had the final say in medical decisions, as long as the attending did not overrule. Each patient was delegated to an intern, who did much of the daily grunt work. Some of the intern's patients were also assigned to a medical student, who usually ended up spending much more time with these patients than any other member of the team.

Because of this, as a third-year student, I was surprised and gratified to learn that many patients considered me to be their "doctor" and referred to me as such. At Georgetown, as is the case at most medical schools, residents and attendings—the real doctors—wore long white coats, while medical students wore shorter white coats. Very few patients, however, realized this subtle distinction or could tell the difference. If we students treated them professionally, they considered us doctors, no matter how we introduced ourselves or what we were wearing.

During the clinical years, my days began early, often at five or six in the morning, depending on how many patients I had to see, with "pre-rounds." This usually involved the thankless task of waking up a sick person who doubtless had trouble sleeping in the hospital and had only just drifted off before you arrived bright and early to interrupt her dreams. After jolting the patient from sleep, I then asked routine questions about her subjective symptoms: Is your pain better or worse? Is the new medication helping your nausea? Are you tolerating the liquid diet? Have you had a bowel movement? Any difficulty urinating?

I then performed a focused physical exam, usually including a quick run through the heart, lungs, abdomen, and a closer look at the patient's particular problems—surgical wounds, rashes, leg swelling, and so forth. The patients often had questions, some of which I could answer, some of which I deferred to the resident. If the questioning went on too long, I would begin to feel restless and simultaneously guilty for feeling so. Pressed for time, I would steal a glance at the clock, trying not to appear hasty, but looking for an opportunity to slip out. My thoughts would inadvertently wander: *I would love to stay, but I have four other patients to see in the next half hour before rounds began, and I already woke up at four-thirty to get here and don't think I can get myself out of bed any earlier, but I hate rushing through in the morning when the patients are looking to me for support, and I hope the attending doesn't ask me about the differential diagnosis for and causes of pancreatitis, since I got home so late last night that I didn't have time to read about it, and I wonder if I have asked the patient all the right questions and looked in all the right orifices this morning because I feel like I have forgotten something, and I'm hungry because there was no time for breakfast, and I forgot to pack a lunch, so hopefully a drug rep will bring food to the noon conference . . .*

A typical 5:30 a.m. conversation would sound something like this:

MRS. SMITH *interrupting student's wandering stream of consciousness*: Doctor, am I going to need surgery?
STUDENT: *Pointing to GoLytely bottle (a misnomer)*: We're not sure yet, Mrs. Smith. We still need to see what the colonoscopy shows. That's scheduled for sometime this morning. Make sure you drink all of the bowel prep stuff in this bottle over the next two hours.
MRS. SMITH: *Wrinkling her nose*: Oh, that stuff puts you on the toilet for hours. I can't stand it. I had to drink that nasty stuff five years ago when I had my last surgery. Hey, I read this article about this new colonoscopy where all you have to do is swallow a tiny pill that actually has a camera in it and the camera takes pictures of your bowel and sends the pictures electronically to this thing you wear on your belt. Do you have that at Georgetown?
STUDENT: No, I'm afraid not. That technology is still in the works. I don't think it's been marketed yet. And it still requires a bowel prep.
MRS. SMITH: Maybe they have a trial up at the NIH; they test lots of new stuff up there, you know. My brother-in-law was in a drug trial there for this new diabetes medication. Stuff made him sick. He dropped out of the trial because of the nasty side effects—constipation, real bad. Maybe you heard about this drug? Starts with a "C" I think, or maybe it was an "S" . . .
STUDENT: *Making his way toward the door*: No, I don't think so. Just be sure to drink the entire bowel-prep bottle . . .

And on to the next patient.

After seeing the patients, it was time to write the notes in the charts. Without fail, the chart rack at the nurses' station somehow contained all the charts on the floor, in exactly the right place, except for the ones I happened to be looking for. After wasting fifteen more precious minutes tracking them down, I would sit down and begin to frantically peruse them. Any new orders since yesterday? Perhaps the intern on call started a new medication or ordered another test. I would glance at the notes written since I left the hospital the day before to see if there were any overnight events the patient failed to tell me about—like the patient falling out of bed, busting his skull, and getting a head CT, the results of which the resident would expect me to know.

STUDENT: You didn't tell me you fell out of bed last night, Mr. Jones.
MR. JONES: Oh, yeah. Forgot about that. You see, I was craning my head to catch a glimpse of that pretty young nurse, when all of a sudden . . .

Now it was time to write my notes, using the conventional "SOAP" format: (1) Subjective: what the patient tells me—complaints or improvements, waxing and waning of symptoms. (2) Objective: the stats, including "vital signs" (temperature, heart rate, blood pressure, respiratory rate, oxygen saturation), fluid "ins & outs" (how many cc's did the patient drink, get via IV or feeding tube; how many cc's did he "put out" in a urine catheter, the toilet, or via surgical drains). The Objective section also contained my physical exam, and the results of any labs, radiological studies, or diagnostic tests. (3) Assessment: the patient's problems, listed numerically if there were a few, or categorized by organ system if there were many. (4) Plan: the most difficult part for a medical student—what to do next, which could include changes in medications, new tests or procedures, discharge from hospital, transfer to another service, and so on. My notes varied in length: up to two or three pages for a medicine patient, usually only half a page for a surgical patient.

Surgeons are notorious for writing the briefest notes. The joke is that the only thing a general surgeon cares about is whether the patient has passed gas—the all-important sign that the gut is working again after abdominal surgery, when it typically shuts down for a time. Only after a surgical patient farts is he given the green light to resume eating, a sure sign that the patient is headed for discharge soon. One surgery resident at Georgetown was famous for the brevity and clarity of his daily progress notes, which usually numbered four to six words. My favorite note of all time was written by this master of simplicity. In large, bold block letters that filled an entire page, it announced triumphantly: "Passed Flatus." Below these two magnificent words, the note was neatly signed and dated, as if to say, "Need I say more?"

On a good day, I would have finished all my notes by the time rounds began. The term "rounds" originated at Johns Hopkins University Hospital: The first hospital building there has a rotunda set underneath a large dome with the patients' rooms arranged in circular fashion around the perimeter. Hence the "residents" (so-called because they actually lived at the hospital) and attendings would literally go "round" to see the patients. According to hospital custom, during rounds, the medical student "presents" his patient to the rest of the team, giving the entire history and full physical exam if the patient was admitted the day prior, or updating the team with a briefer presentation on the daily progress of the patient. The team then discusses the patient and decides on a treatment plan for the day. They visit the patient briefly to double-check the medical student or intern's assessment and to answer further questions the patient may have.

Internal medicine rounds were notoriously long: Every detail was discussed, every possibility considered. Surgical rounds were notoriously short: The surgeon's goal was to get off the "floor" where the patients reside as quickly as possible to get down to the operating room, where he felt most at home. On surgery rounds, efficiency was paramount.

"Miss McCarthy, have you passed gas?"

"No."

"How is your pain?"

"Getting better. Doc, I just have a few quest—"

But it was too late. The surgical team was already in the next room.

The most anxiety-provoking aspect of daily rounds for medical students is the customary questioning by the attending or senior resident, a practice that goes by the infelicitous term "pimping." (I am unaware of the exact origin of this unsavory expression, but you can probably guess the context.) Pimping involves a barrage of increasingly difficult questions, aimed at testing the medical student's "fund of knowledge." Pimp questions range from topics of disease and differential diagnosis to prognosis and pathology. Everything is fair game: obscure physiology, the latest research or study, the history of medicine, medical etymology, or any other trivia—usually, but not necessarily, medical—that the attending deems worthy. When pimped, the student always loses. No matter how many questions the student answers correctly, most attendings do not stop until they have stumped the neophyte. Not even the Gunners can survive a determined Pimper.

The deck is stacked from the beginning: The questioner holds all the cards in his hand. Naturally, he only asks questions to which he knows the answer. On rare occasions, an overachieving medical student may happen to know more details than the attending about the particular topic on which he is being pimped; he may have spent hours the night before reading the latest research. It does not matter; he will still lose. The rules of the game dictate this, because he is only allowed to answer questions, and there is never a shortage of potential questions. If the student is on a roll, the attending may simply decide to change topics, moving on to something the attending knows more about. The Pimpee never gets the opportunity to fire questions back at the Pimper. I have heard stories about imprudent medical students who dug themselves an early grave by asking the attending a pimp question after having answered all the attending's questions correctly. As you can probably surmise, such attempts to one-up a superior do not go over well.

Surgeons sometimes pimp during rounds, but more often, they do this in the operating room. Since surgeons live and breathe anatomy, surgical pimp questions usually follow suit. Questions are invariably anatomical.

"What's this structure?" the surgeon asked me, pointing toward a small strand of white in the otherwise red surgical field.

"That's the ninth cranial nerve—the glossopharyngeal," I replied, relieved to have dodged another bullet.

"Right. What's this?" pointing to a small bleb on a vessel.

"The branch point of the common carotid." Too easy. There must be more coming.

"I mean, what physiological structure is located inside?"

"The carotid body." Getting more nervous.

"Good. What branch of what cranial nerve enervates the carotid body?"

"A branch of the ninth?" I venture, trying to delay the inevitable.

"What's its name?" the surgeon insists, becoming annoyed at my guesswork.

I admit, defeated, "I don't know."

Then came the usual jab—the surgeon's favorite rhetorical question, "Do they still teach gross anatomy in medical school?" Ha, ha.

A study published in the *Journal of the American Medical Association* in 1989 concluded that the practice of pimping suppresses spontaneous or intellectual questions or pursuits, creates an antagonistic atmosphere, and perpetuates medical student abuse.[3] Most medical educators appear to know nothing of this study, however, and the age-old practice of pimping continues.

Rounds were followed by routine patient care: assisting on surgeries; delivering babies; performing bedside procedures, such as a lumbar puncture (a.k.a. spinal tap); thoracentesis (draining fluid off the lungs with a needle); or paracentesis (draining fluid from the abdomen).

Much time was spent tracking down lab results, consulting with other physicians, reading radiological films, writing or dictating discharge summaries, admitting patients, and attending teaching conferences and departmental meetings.

There was also plenty of "scut" work: thankless, boring, and menial tasks, which are only marginally related to patient care and have little educational value. Bad interns scut-out their med students too much, pawning off these jobs on their subordinates: Go fetch this, go tell so-and-so that, go clean up the mess I just made at the bedside, go get me some pizza. Good medical students take on the scut work without being asked. The interns love you for it.

"See one, do one, teach one." This was the basic method for learning bedside procedures. On most days, I would see one; on a good day, I would do one.

My first procedure was a lumbar puncture, a technique used to obtain a sample of cerebrospinal fluid (CSF), the clear broth that bathes the brain and spinal cord. The brain actually floats in this bath of CSF, which cushions it from the surrounding bony skull. CSF samples are often used to diagnose brain disorders, especially infections in or around the brain. To obtain a small sample of this precious liquid, the physician must blindly navigate a long needle through the bony lumbar spine, puncture the tough dural sac that surrounds the spinal cord, and stop in the small space that houses the CSF, allowing this special juice to drain drop by drop into a vial. The body, in her wisdom, guards the spinal cord carefully, situating it within a fortress of vertebral bones and ligaments. Access is granted only to the careful navigator of the needle.

For the procedure, the patient lay on her side, curled in a fetal position, her back toward me. Over her back was a sterile drape, with a space open at the puncture site, which I had cleaned with betadine solution. I stood gowned and gloved in sterile fashion, holding a small bottle of local anesthetic.

"This is the worst part," I told her, stretching the truth a bit. "I'm going to inject some numbing medication." I depressed the syringe, and watched as the skin rose in a "wheel," the lidocaine dispersing in the subcutaneous space. The feel of a needle in my hand was not entirely new, as I had already drawn plenty of blood on my psychiatry rotation. The phlebotomists refused to come onto the locked psych ward to stick psychotic patients with needles (one can hardly blame them), so naturally the task of drawing blood there was delegated to the medical students. Prior to injecting this lidocaine, I had always used needles to take something from the patient. Now I was dispensing something into the patient, a substance that would inactivate the nerves responsible for carrying pain signals.

With the area over the spine sufficiently numb, it was time to uncork the larger needle. With my fingers, I tried to feel the anatomical landmarks—the bony spinous processes at the third and fourth lumbar vertebrae, the iliac crest laterally. Feigning confidence in my voice, I tried to reassure the patient, as though I had done this plenty of times before: "Don't worry, this won't take long." The resident stood by, instructing me in whispered tones. I did not tell the patient that I was a lumbar puncture virgin—that this was my first time.

This procedure is usually mildly traumatic: One typically obtains a bit of blood mixed in with the CSF. After sending the sample off to the lab, the student waits to see the results appear on the computer. Of course, he wants to see the test results that relate to the patient's diagnosis. He also, however, is interested in the number of red blood cells (RBCs) in the sample. The perfect tap—a rare occurrence—has none. Zero RBCs, the coveted "champagne tap," is named after a venerated tradition: The intern or student who performs the perfect tap is treated to a bottle of champagne, courtesy of his senior resident or attending.

Desiring victory, I took aim. I advanced the needle, stopped, and pulled back on the plunger, hoping to see clear fluid. There was none.

Undeterred, I advanced again, hit bone, withdrew, changed directions ever so slightly, and continued. Deeper the needle went, disappearing further into the patient's back. Without warning, she suddenly cried out in pain and tensed up. I winced. "Sorry. I'm going to give you some more numbing medication." More lidocaine, deeper this time, then back in with the large needle. Still no fluid. I began to perspire under the sterile gown.

After a seemingly interminable period, the resident took over. I sighed, both disappointed and relieved. In seconds, the resident's deft fingers had the invading needle inside the spinal fortress, and the prized fluid was dripping out the other end. "Don't worry, you'll get it next time," she said.

See one, do one, teach one. At that point, I was still stuck on the second step.

The culture of medicine, which I became fully exposed to during these clinical years, exerted subtle effects on my demeanor. No medical student is immune from these influences; if one is not careful, they may shape him in ways that he would not have chosen. A particularly pernicious effect I noticed was this: Manners tend to become coarsened. In a hospital, everyone is in a constant hurry; formalities are thus dispensed with. No one has time. Efficiency is king. Social niceties take time, so different rules of etiquette apply.

One day, I was discussing this phenomenon with a psychiatry resident, who had pointed out that no one in the hospital bothers to address you by your name. A moment later, a social worker burst into his office, and without so much as an "excuse me, Doctor," interrupted our conversation and began complaining to him about something or another relating to his patient. He looked at me, and gave a knowing smile, as if to say, "See what I mean?"

Residents do not answer pages with, "Hello, this is Dr. Kheriaty answering a page," but with, "Yeah?" This is, after all, much more efficient. Too much cordiality or politeness actually annoys many residents. There were some attendings I worked under who never bothered to introduce themselves or ask my name. When consulting a resident on another service, if my explanation included any unnecessary words or what they considered irrelevant facts, they gave me an exasperated why-are-you-wasting-my-time-hurry-up-and-get-to-the-point look.

Such is the anemic culture of medicine. No wasted time. No wasted words. No wasted energy. No polite trivialities. All business. Keep up the pace.

For most initiates, it is no exaggeration to say that the hospital is unlike anything they have ever encountered. It is, quite literally, a different world.

The philosopher Martin Heidegger drew a distinction between a person's "environment" and a person's "world." One's environment consists of all that one is surrounded by—the totality of one's sensory input and experience. One's world is a smaller subset of one's environment and consists of all the things in the environment for which the person knows the name. The act of naming a thing, or of learning its name, brings the thing from one's environment into one's world. Because he alone among all the animals has the capacity for language, man is the only animal that lives in a world; the other animals merely exist in an environment. This is symbolized by Adam naming the animals in the Garden of Eden. The late novelist Walker Percy added an interesting twist when he observed that what Sigmund Freud called the "unconscious" can be understood as all the things in one's environment that one has experienced but has not yet named—things that are therefore not yet a part of his conscious world.

The new third-year student, when he steps into the hospital, enters a new environment. Only after he learns the language and local customs does this foreign environment become his native world. As he learns the strange names, the peculiar jargon—in short, as he learns the language and begins to speak it—he soon begins to feel more at home in this new world.

So immersed do some doctors become in the world of medicine that they seem forget their native tongue. They often have difficulty translating medical jargon back into language their patients can understand, despite having once spoken this language themselves. It is a strange phenomenon: to see a highly educated physician who cannot refrain from using medical terminology, while the hapless patient tries in vain to comprehend what the doctor is saying. The strange language of medicine serves to alienate the patient.

The new language of medicine produces new patterns of thought. Take, as one example among many, the way physicians (and medical students) speak about sex. They engage in what I call the sterilization of the erotic. Our profession requires us to behave as though it were perfectly natural to ask our patients about this intimate mystery in the same breath that we inquire about their bowel habits. To get around this, we attempt to create a sterile field around sex, placing it under the fluorescent lights of our clinics.

During our first two years of medical school, we were instructed on numerous occasions to get accustomed to talking about sex with our patients. We learned to be matter-of-fact, to avoid the supposedly childish blush. While this tactic is certainly necessary to gather relevant clinical data, the danger is that we will get used to speaking (and therefore, thinking) of sex as though it were merely one more physiological process. The language we use to talk about sex changes the way we think about sex. As one of the most influential philosophers of the twentieth century, Ludwig Wittgenstein, said, "The limits of my language are the limits of my world."[4]

What words are available to the physician, who must daily tread such dangerous ground? A former college professor of mine, David O'Conner, in a brilliant essay to which I am indebted here, argues that the worst terms are those we doctors employ in the clinic. The impoverishment of our language of love came initially from talk of "safe sex" that started under the influence of the public health authorities. O'Conner has this to say about this medical turn in our language of love—what he calls a "prophylactic of the tongue":

> "Sexual intercourse" comes from the same region of the language native to various sorts of -ectomies and -oscopies. It does not sound like something for which one would cross the hall, let alone the world. "I'm sorry, I can't meet you for lunch today; I have to go to the medical center for a sexual intercourse." My favorite illustration of where this way of talking takes us is the phrase "sexually active." It seems to be modeled on "radioactive": the "sexually active" teenager is an isotope with a short half-life, spewing particles of sexuality that threaten to cause beta decay in the surrounding atoms.[5]

I am here reminded of the psychiatrist's constant recourse to the equally silly term "sex life," which is often spoken of as though one were asking the patient, "So, how's your golf game?" Such questioning usually provokes responses that mirror the golf analogy—something to the effect of, "Well, I'm a bit out of practice," or "Pretty good, I've played eighteen holes a few times already this week." Another favorite clinical question is asking about the number of sexual "partners," a term that, for some reason, reminds me of tennis partners—sex as intimate mystery becomes sex as sport. O'Connor concludes, "The metallic aftertaste of words medical and the impudent tastelessness of words adolescent make every choice unpalatable."[6]

All of medicine's efforts at taming Eros, whether through language, latex, or countless mechanical-hormonal devices, have failed. Love is never tamed; sex is never safe. Our attempts to create a sterile field around it are useless. The sterilizing sponges of our medical jargon, ceaselessly scrubbed into our minds, are insufficient. Love and sex remain forever beyond our impoverished clinical words. Therefore, physicians should approach this topic with a degree of awe, even of reverential fear. We need to learn to tread lightly, even as we employ language that is sterile and cumbersome.

Sacred language—"nuptial meaning of the body," "conjugal embrace," and the like—while unlikely to make its way into the everyday lexicon or the physician's jargon, can serve to remind doctors of what their clinical language causes them to forget. After taking countless sexual histories, after performing innumerable pelvic exams, it is well for the physician to be reminded that at the deepest level, sex is more than plumbing, more than the movement of fluids. Elevated language is, however, foreign to medicine's usual linguistic atmosphere. To claim sex as something special, much less something sacred, as something fundamentally different from other biological processes—to so much as hint at its mystery—invites ridicule.

I am not arguing that physicians should change our medical terminology; such a solution, even if possible, would be doomed to failure. After importing language more equal to the subject, the sacred vocabulary would rapidly become profane through routine clinical use. Instead, as physicians who must inevitably employ the detached language of clinicians, we must remain aware of the inherent dangers. We must be on guard, lest the banality of our reductive terminology completely anesthetize our thinking.

Human aspirations stretch further than our language. Clinical language diminishes the highest things. Therefore, I urge my fellow physicians: Let not the limits of our language be the limits of our world.

This clinical, objectifying language also distances physicians from patients' everyday experience of health and illness. It is designed, in part, to do just this. Clinical distance is sometimes necessary for objectivity, but too much arbitrary separation removes the physician from the realities of the illnesses they treat. Taken to excess, the language barrier separates physician and patient. Søren Kierkegaard was aware of the danger of impersonal functionalism, where a man is so entirely absorbed in his role that he loses his humanity. A doctor should be a man before he is a doctor.

Objectifying clinical language fashions the doctor into "a biological accountant engaged in input/output calculations."[7] This perfectly describes what I often felt like as a third-year clerk. As philosopher and social critic Ivan Illich explains, with the detached language of the clinic, the patient's experience of sickness is "taken from him and turned into the raw material for an institutional enterprise." In this process of expropriation, the patient's condition is "interpreted according to a set of abstract rules in a language he cannot understand. He is taught about alien entities that the doctor combats, but only just as much as the doctor considers necessary to gain the patient's cooperation."[8]

The patient is left mystified when all language used to describe his condition is taken over by the medical experts with their technical jargon: "The sick person is deprived of meaningful words for his anguish, which is thus further increased by linguistic mystification." Illich explains, by contrast, "Before scientific slang had come to dominate language about the body, the repertory of ordinary speech in this field was exceptionally rich." This mystifying language results a class-based system of exclusion and unintentional punching down: "The university-trained and the bureaucrat thus become their doctor's colleague in the treatment he dispenses, while the worker is put in his place as a subject who does not speak the language of his master."[9]

Medical practitioners starting in the late nineteenth century produced our current system of mystifying knowledge when they decided they must think and talk like scientists at the bedside. Doctors must not only be trained in anatomy, physiology, pathology, virology, pharmacology, and so forth; they must also conceptualize diseases exclusively in terms of micro-concepts of cellular pathology, bacteriology, and so forth.[10] This led to medical specialization, eventually resulting in today's hyper-specialization. This push toward greater specialization rests upon a reductionist analysis of the body and disease—the assumption that each organ or organ system operates in relative isolation from the whole.

When I first arrived on the wards, I was astonished to see patients with a dozen different diagnoses on their "problem list," each of which was dealt with separately during treatment planning. It made no sense that a patient could have so many different derangements in so many different organ systems. How could one patient be so unlucky, afflicted by so many different diseases? The answer is that they were not really distinct diseases: These disparate problems must have had deeper underlying causes knitting them together. But we rarely explored those deeper causes, preferring a symptom-management approach that applied a new drug or procedure for every symptom or syndrome.

A person with nine different symptoms or problems most likely does not need to see nine different specialists who will each apply a specific remedy to the respective organ system—the internist for obesity and hypertension, the nephrologist for kidney dysfunction, the endocrinologist for diabetes, the psychiatrist for depression or early dementia, and the infectious disease doctor for immune system malfunctions. These are likely not disconnected problems, but diverse manifestations of underlying metabolic derangements caused by modifiable dietary and environmental toxicities. If none of the specialists examines those underlying issues, the patient ends up on a dozen different medications, many of them for life, and subjected to half a dozen procedures. Once you get on this treatment treadmill, it's hard to get off. The expansionist medical empire grows, and big pharma rakes in profits, but our overall health continues to decline.

By contrast, traditional Hippocratic medicine thought of health and disease holistically, in terms of the general relationship between bodily systems or between the person and the environment. While scientific knowledge was admittedly primitive, the philosophy emphasized dietetics and environmental factors influencing health and illness. The Hippocratic physician attempted to understand the body as a whole and see the patient as existing in a social and environmental context. Drugs had an ancillary role, and surgery was to be done by specialists only very judiciously. Advances in pharmacology and surgery have clearly made them more attractive options, but the underlying Hippocratic philosophy of medicine still has much to teach us. Effectiveness in managing symptoms in isolation from the whole has not led to beneficial overall health outcomes.

Hyper-specialized medical imperialism metastasizes in other ways as well, invading aspects of everyday life that were not previously subject to medical management or control. As medicine becomes an increasingly pervasive social force, the language of the clinic tends to seep out into other sectors of society. Various individual and social problems—political and moral—become medicalized, recast in the language of the clinic. The last several decades have seen the rise of what sociologist Philip Rieff called the triumph of the therapeutic. Nonmedical issues—from criminality and deviance to shyness and short stature—come to be defined, and often treated, as medical problems.

The profound consequences of medicalization include, among other things, the loss of a sense of personal agency. If, for example, obesity is primarily a medical problem—rather than a behavioral, environmental, societal, or lifestyle problem—then one is powerless to address it without the prescription from a doctor, the sole gatekeeper to better health. To take another example, many parents feel disempowered to raise children without the expert advice of pediatricians or child psychologists at every stage of development. Complex human problems are reduced to one-dimensional medical issues, and rich sources of wisdom for living and flourishing are discarded or ignored. This kind of medicalization is profitable, however: A recent study of "disease mongering"—widening the boundaries of treatable illness in order to expand markets for those who sell and deliver treatments—demonstrates how pharmaceutical companies sponsor diseases and promote them to prescribers and consumers.[11]

We have always ritualized certain stages of life, but now we medicalize them, from menarche and menopause to aging and death. But unlike the rituals of old, which may have been intense but were time-limited, the post-menopausal medical interventions continue indefinitely under medical supervision in the modern cathedral of the hospital or clinic—the new archetypal institution of Western culture. Unborn children are medically surveilled and frequently eliminated when found to be defective according to our quality-control metrics. We turn perfectly healthy newborns into hospitalized patients until they are medicated, vaccinated, and certified healthy. The public is fascinated by high tech care, mesmerized by claims of chemically engineered miracles.

"Intensive care is but the culmination of a public worship organized around a medical priesthood struggling against death,"[12] in Ivan Illich's vivid description. As we will explore in the next chapter, perhaps more thoroughly than any other feature of human life, even death has been medicalized. "Through the medicalization of death, health care has become a monolithic world religion. . . . In its extreme form, 'natural death' is now that point at which the human organism refuses any further input of treatment." Indeed, in Illich's description, "The medicalization of society has brought the epoch of natural death to an end. Western man has lost the right to preside at his act of dying."[13]

CHAPTER 4

Their Exits and Their Entrances

The last act is bloody, however fine the rest of the play.
They throw earth over your head and it is finished forever.
—Blaise Pascal, *Pensées*[1]

The last act—death—is bloody. So too is the first act—birth. We make our entrance on the world's stage squealing and covered in sanguineous slime. Echoing the metaphor of life as theatrical drama, the Bard gave us the famous lines, "All the world's a stage, and all the men and women merely players; they have their exits and their entrances."[2] And for better or worse, these exits and entrances happen today most often in our hospitals, with the doctor as a kind of director ushering players on and off the stage.

The first act is indeed bloody, but also beautiful. It is an astonishing experience to have the first hands to touch a newborn human being, to grip him while he is still emerging from the body of his mother. You hold his bloody little body and don't let him go as you usher him into the world. He opens his eyes, and you are the first person he ever sees.

The labor and delivery service on my obstetrics clerkship initially frustrated me. All my patients seemed to end up having cesareans. After wresting away responsibility for births from midwives in the twentieth century and removing childbirth from the home to the hospital, obstetrics has become trigger-happy—too eager to slice open expectant mothers to expedite delivery. Medicalized childbirth introduces constant monitoring, which increases the impulse to intervene and hurry the delivery process to completion. Waiting patiently is harder when alarm bells are buzzing and the mom is experiencing labor-related distress.

Maternal mortality has dropped with modern interventional obstetrics, surely a great blessing, but at the cost of unnecessary interventions with their own set of complications. The World Health Organization considers the ideal rate for C-section births to be between 10 percent and 15 percent for optimizing maternal health outcomes.[3] However, the CDC reports that 32 percent of all deliveries in the United States in 2022 were by C-section, more than double the recommended rate.[4] According to the WHO, "non-clinical factors such as women increasingly wanting to determine how and when their child is born, generational shifts in work and family responsibilities, physician factors including increasing fear of medical litigation, as well as organizational, economic and social factors have all been implicated in this increase."[5] Notice that medical justifications—maternal or infant morbidity and mortality—are not included on this list.

Consistent with this trend, my first several patients on the labor and delivery service went to the operating room for delivery. Not that this method of delivery was unimpressive or lacked interest for the medical student. But I'd already completed my surgery rotation and was eager to deliver a baby with my own two hands instead of just holding the retractors on a cesarean while the resident or attending lifted the newborn baby out of the spliced-open womb.

As students, we had practiced delivery using little floppy dolls. We learned how to maneuver the head to allow the shoulders through, how to grip the back of the neck firmly but not too tight, how to slide the other hand down the back and buttocks, and how to get a firm hold of the thigh so as not to drop the baby once it fully emerged.

"They're slippery, just like they look. If you've got a tight grip on the leg, even if you lose your hold on top, you won't drop it," the resident explained. "You see, your hand always stops sliding at the ankle," he said as he held up the doll upside-down by the leg. I pictured a horrified mother looking on as I dangled her baby by the ankle. *Let's try to avoid that.*

As I prepared for my first vaginal delivery, I looked down below the patient and noticed a plastic bag opened on the ground—but no safety net. For some reason, I had expected one. I mean, why not? The baby's skin was, as the resident had warned, surprisingly slippery. The plastic bag rested on the hard floor and would not cushion the baby in the event of a fall. (I'd never heard of a medical student dropping a baby during delivery but didn't want to be the pioneer on this.) The resident had assured me there would be other hands to help. There were none: They let me catch the baby on my own. I had to scramble to catch him in time.

I had been in the labor and delivery room with the patient for some time, coaching her through the contractions, periodically checking the dilation of her cervix, and trying to reassure her and the father that things were progressing well. When I could see the crown of the baby's head, I notified the resident, who went to page the attending. They both arrived ready in gown and sterile gloves. By contrast, I was still wearing scrubs, not dressed for the possibility of a gush of body fluids when the baby came out.

"If you want to do this," said the attending, "you'd better gown up quick."

I scrambled around the room, checking the drawers and kicking myself for not getting my sterile items out earlier. After what seemed like an age, a nurse handed me a gown. I fumbled with the ties, donned the mask, and snapped a fresh pair of gloves on my sweaty palms.

A few seconds later, the baby's head emerged. He was facing down, and I knew that his head would have to turn, either toward his mother's right leg or her left, so that he faced forward (babies come out "sideways," so to speak). I did not know which way to turn the head, and I did not want to twist it backward! Fortunately, the baby did it for me—turning toward the right leg.

With one hand over each of his ears, I gently pushed the head down toward the floor, and his left shoulder popped out. I then pulled his head up toward the ceiling, and his right shoulder followed. The rest of his body slid out easily. Suddenly, he was free in my hands, attached to his mother's body only by the gooey cord from his belly. To my relief, I neither dangled nor dropped him. My hands grasped—firmly but not too tight—the gooey little boy. A nurse clamped and cut the cord as I held him close.

During all this, I had become almost completely unaware of other sights and sounds around me—a psychological phenomenon known as dissociation. I looked down at the newborn's tiny body, coated in gray mucous and wriggling in my white gloves. His eyes opened, and he took his first look at the world outside the womb. The baby's mother, wholly spent, looked at her son for the first time. Then at me. I placed the child on her chest. She cradled him and smiled in silence. I stood dumbstruck for a moment, motionless. For a time, the clocks all froze.

The bustle of nurses, the chatter of doctors, the cooing of proud new parents. My tunnel-vision meant I had taken in little of this until I delivered this tiny boy. Now those sounds and sights returned as I regained my senses.

The "miracle" of childbirth has become a shopworn cliché. But how else can we describe this event, so charged with mystery and meaning, the experience of all human experiences? What can we say of this separate and distinct new one emerging fresh from the dark warmth of the female body? Poet Matthias Claudius, in "The human being," presents our entrance on the stage in unadorned lines:

> *Received and nurtured*
> *of woman wonderful,*
> *he comes and sees and hears*
> *and does not perceive the deceit* . . .[6]

The child I delivered did not, for example, perceive that I had no idea what I was doing: "Hey there, kid. Welcome to the world. Yes, this was my first time ushering a player onto the world-stage. Glad you made it here okay." He did, however, perceive my astonished gaze. And I perceived him. Indeed, he was the *only* thing I could perceive in that moment. Everything else faded. To this day, more than twenty years later, I can picture his face though I do not recall his name.

I never saw him again. There is only one thing I know with certainty about that child: Someday he will die. And odds are he will again be under the care of a physician when that happens. After describing the newborn's growth through the stages of life, Claudius's poem concludes with these lines:

*and all this lasts
if it gets high, eighty years.
Then he lies down with his fathers,
and he never comes back.*[7]

We are, as it were, born towards dying. "They give birth astride of a grave," Samuel Beckett wrote in *Waiting for Godot*, "the light gleams an instant, then it's night once more."[8]

Biology is defined as the study of living things—*bio-logos*—the study of life. But biologists have a notoriously difficult time defining life itself. We have yet to formulate a clear definition which includes all living things and excludes all non-living things. Everyone seems to recognize life when they see it. We all share some intuition about what life is and is not. Nonetheless, strange to say, a concise scientific definition still eludes us. In their attempts, biologists typically resort to listing certain properties supposedly found among all living things, such as organization, growth, metabolism, adaptation, reproduction, and so on. They debate about this or that item on the list and come up with apparent counterexamples to some items to be found among very small, strange, or obscure organisms.

Biologists ignore, in my opinion, one simple definition: A living organism is something that can and will die. Some may object that this "definition" is a tautology or a truism—that it elucidates nothing. If it is a truism, then it is a profound one. Defining life as that which is mortal or "death-able" tells us a great deal about it. In the case of living human beings, it reminds us of something we often prefer to forget, deny, or ignore. Death is inexorably bound up with life. You cannot have one without the other. "In the midst of life we are in death," in the words of a medieval Latin antiphon.[9]

Death is not something the physician can ignore, even if we take pains to avoid it. Doctors are constantly surrounded by death. It's not that every patient under one's care will die while in treatment. The point is rather that every diseased organ, every broken body part, every new ailment, is a proleptic sign—a reminder—of the patient's mortality. So death is ever-present in medicine, even if it often only lurks in the background.

Doctors frequently see death as their ultimate enemy, even if unconsciously. But this is a mistake—a "fatal" mistake, if you'll excuse the pun. Because if the last enemy is death, then doctors are playing a losing-game in every case. If our goal is the conquest of death, then the physician is engaged in a futile exercise, the outcome of which is predetermined, and all his efforts are in vain.

Medicine's true goal must be more modest: health and life, but not perfect health or eternal life. The health he promotes, the life he preserves, is always finite, always destined ultimately for the grave. In the midst of life, we are in death. As Paul Ramsey, one of the founding fathers of American bioethics, put it in his classic work *The Patient as Person*, "Doctors do not treat diseases, though they often conquer them. They treat patients, and here finally all fail."[10]

"Where are you going?" I asked the medical resident on call one evening. "I thought we were grabbing dinner from the cafeteria."

"I know," she replied. "But I just got paged. I've got to take care of something real quick. I'll meet you there in ten minutes."

"Do you need help?"

"No, thanks, I'll take care of this one. I have to go declare a patient."

I wondered for a second: *You need to declare a patient what? Declare something to a patient? Tell a patient what?* No, I heard her correctly: "declare a patient." She avoided saying that she had to declare a patient *dead*. This was my first clue that there was a word physicians almost never used. In fact, they often played elaborate language games to avoid mentioning it.

Not long after that, during morning rounds, I noticed that a patient who had been on our service the day before had disappeared. I didn't think there had been plans to discharge him, so I asked, "What happened to Mr. James?" Matter-of-factly, the resident said, "He expired last night." I was puzzled. "He . . . *expired?*" Coupons expire. Milk expires. People *die*. There it was again—the D-word, studiously elided with a weird euphemism.

It's not just doctors who avoid the subject. We live in a death-denying society, as cultural anthropologist Ernest Becker explained fifty years ago in his Pulitzer Prize–winning book, *The Denial of Death*. Becker noted that the human animal is characterized by two great fears that other animals are spared—the fear of life and the fear of death. "The irony of man's condition is that the deepest need is to be free of the anxiety of death and annihilation; but it is life itself which awakens it, and so we must shrink from being fully alive."[11] Becker argued that the denial of death was the central driving force shaping contemporary society and human behavior. He believed that the modern age has lost the cultural and religious resources to deal with death, so we repress thoughts about our mortality. But as the psychoanalysts taught us, that which we repress does not thereby disappear; it returns in the form of personal neuroses and cultural pathologies. Death still haunts a death-denying culture. And it haunts a death-denying medical system.

We can try to avoid it. We can deny it. But we can't ultimately escape it. Medicine will continue to improve over the next fifty years—new cures, better surgical techniques, therapies we haven't yet imagined. But I hope that the biggest advances will emerge in our ability to accept medicine's limitations. Death represents the unsurpassable horizon against which we practice medicine. The futile attempt to defeat death through biomedical science—the dream of the transhumanist movement—will only result in undermining our humanity.

Despite the salutary rise of palliative care as a specialty, most doctors still have not learned to help patients die well. The rise of palliative care is in fact a symptom of the problem, even if it also forms part of the needed solution. That we need a specialty to do what all doctors should be trained to do is not a sign of medicine's health. The necessary medical advance I am advocating—the acceptance of our mortality—will not come as a technical solution to a scientific problem. Scientific research and public funding will not help. The necessary advance will have to be a more humane approach to the deep mystery of every mortal human life. Medicine needs to learn to do less, not more—to step aside with humility and a sense of its inherent limits.

The movement to legalize physician-assisted suicide and euthanasia is another symptom of the current problems that plague end-of-life medical care. On the surface, allowing doctor-assisted suicide might seem like a step toward accepting our mortality: When a cure is not possible, we can embrace death on our own terms. But this proposed "solution" is really just another form of denial. It solves nothing, because it is premised on the patently false assumption that our autonomy has no inherent limits. It rests upon the delusion that even death can be subject to medical or technocratic control.

Ironically, death is the one event in life which hammers home our lack of ultimate mastery. We did not choose to be born—we are thrown into the world, without being asked, as the philosopher Martin Heidegger put it—nor do we choose whether we die. These basic facts of existence suggest that we are not the sole author of the story of our lives, or of our deaths. Our denial of death manifests in our approach to end-of-life care—at least, in practices that refuse to respect medicine's inherent limitations.

On the one hand, we have the assisted suicide or euthanasia model, which has gained ground in many states and has been enthusiastically embraced in Canada. This is an attempt to completely control the circumstances of one's death through the ingestion or injection of a deadly drug at a time of one's choosing.

On the other hand, we have the more common but likewise futile attempt to continue non-beneficial aggressive treatment at the end-of-life, which only prolongs the dying process without providing meaningful recovery. The machinery of medicine has a momentum of its own, often prolonging life in a state that few people would want—and yet we have a difficult time preventing this outcome or taking the off-ramp. Let's call this misguided approach "therapeutic obstinacy."

Though it may seem paradoxical, active euthanasia and therapeutic obstinacy form flipsides of the same counterfeit coin: Both are a form of medicine's death-denying tendencies. Death cannot finally be brought under rationalized medical control, however hard we try. Our attempts to medically "manage" death are bound to be dehumanizing, even cruel.

Doctors—indeed, our entire society—must learn to allow natural death without becoming the agents of death. Providing all patients access to good palliative care at the end of life is necessary but not sufficient. It's only a starting point. We need also to relearn what used to be called the *ars moriendi*—the art of dying. This involves much more than a morphine for our pain or a sedative to calm our agitation.

It means the opportunity for a person to rectify past wrongs, to reconcile broken relationships, to reorient his or her priorities—to say and to do what really matters most in the end. The art of dying makes space for the really hard conversations: "Please forgive me," "I forgive you," "Thank you," "I love you"—what palliative care physician Ira Byock calls the four things that matter most.[12] Most people today say they want to die at home, but most end up dying in a hospital, many of them in the ICU. Modern medicine has sanitized death, removing it from the lived, communal experience of home, families, and neighbors. This makes saying and doing what matters most in the end more difficult.

The art of dying also involves making space for dying persons to face themselves and come to terms with their lives, including accepting the inevitable missed opportunities and failures—as the protagonist in Leo Tolstoy's famous novella *The Death of Ivan Ilyich* had to do in the process of his decline toward death. The hardest thing for most of us to do might be to look in the mirror, to really look. But knowledge of one's impending death presents a unique opportunity that is not present to the same degree in other stages of life. "Depend upon it, sir," Samuel Johnson remarked to James Boswell, "when a man knows he is to be hanged in a fortnight, it concentrates his mind wonderfully."[13]

But medicine often inhibits this—it pulls the mirror away, as it were—when it offers either assisted suicide or therapeutic obstinacy. These conversations, and the associated interior struggle to contend with life's terminus, are shoved aside to search for the next medical intervention. Our attention shifts to an obsessive focus on lab values, vital signs, or ventilator settings; we defer to the self-perpetuating machinery of the ICU. Meanwhile, the patient declines inevitably toward death in spite of all this. Medicine thereby engages in a form of theft, really—stealing opportunities from vulnerable patients, opportunities that they will never get back.

Watching a loved one die can be incredibly anguishing. But those who have died well show us that in the midst of suffering and decline, we can still find courage, transcendent hope, and even beauty. True compassion and mercy involve walking this difficult journey with our patients and with our loved ones—a journey in which there are no shortcuts. Granted, not everyone can have a death like this. But when the end is foreseeable, medicine can be of assistance in many meaningful ways, but most often by simply getting out of the way. Medical hubris resists admitting these limits. But false medical hope is another form of despair.

What does the medical team do after the resident declares one of their patients dead? They cross the patient off their list. Literally. There's no time for mourning on the wards. Occasionally, I glimpsed tears welling up in someone's eyes or caught a note of sadness in their voice. But this rarely lasted more than a fleeting moment. If a doctor is to go on, his grieving cannot persist long. To an observer, it may appear as though death simply becomes part of the routine. That's what doctors want you to think, at least. Another day, another "expired" patient.

"What doctors *want* you to think" . . . Because there's usually more happening beneath the surface. Working in the presence of death, even if it is not the death of a loved one, weighs on the soul. Yet during my time in medical school, death was never discussed. It was taboo. Why? Perhaps because of death's mystery? The most important things in life are the hardest things to say—words seem to diminish them. Talking of such things leaves us vulnerable, and we prefer silence to stammering.

How did the other doctors deal with death? As a medical student, I could not say. As a believer in God's providence, when confronted by death, I tried to trust his wisdom. "Though he slay me, yet will I hope in him," said Job.[14] Faith does not remove the mystery; it deepens it. I never spoke to anyone about my religious convictions, and no one ever asked about them. In the vicinity of death, the doctors I encountered in medical school established a conspiracy of silence. Each of us was alone with our private experiences. Perhaps in a culture without shared metaphysical convictions or moral frameworks, this is the best we can do. But it's not much good. I'm not even sure it's sustainable.

Mr. Jameson was a forty-eight-year-old male with a one-month history of expressive aphasia (difficulty speaking due to damage of the language center in the brain), ataxia (difficulty walking), hemiparesis (weakness of the right arm and leg), left-sided intermittent headaches for three days, and new-onset urinary retention. The prior week, he had also developed difficulty reading and was seen by an ophthalmologist who said his vision was normal. Since the patient was unable to communicate due to his aphasia, his wife had related this history to me in the emergency room.

His symptoms of weakness in his right arm and leg had begun about three months prior to the present hospital admission. At that time, he had been admitted to the same hospital, and the old records showed that he had received a complete but inconclusive neurological workup. Every possible diagnosis we could think of, from the obvious hypothesis of a stroke down to the most obscure and unlikely cause, had already been considered. Now he was back, his symptoms worsening, and we were no closer to having a firm diagnosis. In the emergency room, we had first considered the possibility of a left-sided stroke, which could have accounted for his right-sided weakness and his aphasia, and possibly his visual changes if the stroke was large enough, but we quickly ruled this out with a head CT. Furthermore, a single stroke could not have been responsible for his urinary retention and ataxia.

I had noticed one other minor finding on the physical exam, which I pointed out to the resident that night. It had not seemed very important at the time, but it later proved decisive. Mr. Jameson had a very subtle rash on his legs: a few scattered dots slightly pinker than the surrounding skin, with a white central clearing, no larger than half a centimeter in diameter. As we sat in teaching rounds scratching our heads, I mentioned the rash once again. The resident picked up a dermatology atlas and began to absently thumb through it. Suddenly, she interrupted the conversation.

"Look at this picture. That's it. That's his rash! Degos disease."

"Never heard of it," the attending said.

"Also called Malignant Atrophic Papulosis. Very rare multi-organ disease . . . a vasculitis, cause is unknown, possibly virally mediated . . . neurologic manifestations in 20 percent of patients, including hemiparesis and aphasia, cranial nerve involvement . . . discovered by Degos in 1942 . . . wow, only 159 reported cases since then. It says that the histology of the rash is diagnostic: We need a skin biopsy."

The left-sided weakness, the headaches, the aphasia, the urinary problems, the intermittent visual disturbances—this single disease could account for all Mr. Jameson's weirdly disparate symptoms. Could the rash be the key that unlocked this diagnostic mystery?

It was a long shot: Degos disease was what we call a "zebra." The old joke goes that when a medical student hears the sound of hoofbeats behind him, the first thing he suspects is not the more obvious horse but the less obvious zebra. Inexperienced medical students have a tendency to think of the most obscure and unlikely diseases when presented with symptoms and asked to come up with a "differential diagnosis." Rare things happen rarely: One almost never turns around and sees a zebra when there are hoofbeats. (In South Africa, where zebras are much more common, the word "canary" is substituted among medical educators.)

We immediately consulted the dermatologist for a biopsy. The results were affirmative: Degos disease. "Great job with the diagnosis," the dermatologist wrote in the chart, congratulating us on identifying the zebra. Our excitement over having nailed the exceptionally rare diagnosis was tempered by what we learned of Mr. Jameson's prognosis. The outlook was very poor for this man who was not yet fifty. According to the textbook we had consulted on rounds, there were no effective treatments. The published cases showed a few instances of spontaneous recovery, but the disease was nearly always lethal.

It was time to tell the patient.

"Mr. Jameson, we figured out what is going on. Your condition is called Degos disease. Unfortunately, there are no known treatments. It tends to be progressive. I'm afraid the news is not good. You probably do not have very long to live. We will have the palliative care team come and see you to talk about your options."

Doctors have these conversations like they are reading from a script. Even the most compassionate and humane doctors have a stock of words and phrases they reach for in these moments. It's hard to make it up as you go along, hard to find the right words for each patient. Maybe because there are no right words.

In this case, the news seemed to register with his wife but not with the patient himself. He continued smiling. This was likely due to the effects on the brain of the illness itself. Our original suspicion of a stroke had not been far off in this sense: Degos disease causes "micro-infarcts" in the brain: mini-strokes that are too small to appear on an MRI or CT, but cumulatively cause neurologic symptoms. Perhaps the damage to his brain was causing a mild dementia, preventing him from really comprehending his situation. This could account for his incongruous smiles in the face of almost certain death.

I stopped at the Georgetown library on my way home. The information we had read on the disease was a few years old, and I wanted to see what had been published in the medical literature since. I found a few more case reports in various journals. Some patients had recovered fully with treatments that were little more than an educated shot-in-the-dark. I paged the resident.

"I did some more research on Degos disease. There is a report of a woman who recovered after anti-platelet therapy," I told her. "It seems reasonable, since this might help prevent the micro-infarcts."

"Great. I'll put him on Plavix."

This is what we do when there is nothing left to do. We try something, whether for ourselves or for the patient or their family is hard to say. This medication was not enough. The day we made the diagnosis was my last day on the service. I never saw Mr. Jameson again. The email from the intern came a few weeks later: Mr. Jameson had died. An interesting "case," everyone had called him. Now he was gone. The zebra had killed him.

Washington, DC. September 11, 2001. I was on neurology rounds at the Washington Veterans Administration Medical Center in the nation's capital. Suddenly, the usual busy activity on the wards slowed to a halt. The staff began turning their attention to the television sets in the patients' rooms. We watched as the World Trade Center towers collapsed. Shortly after, while looking out the window, I could see the black smoke rising from the Pentagon across town.

Every patient in the hospital was a veteran, many of whom had served in World War II. Sick and incapacitated, they watched helplessly as the country they had fought to defend once again came under siege.

I called my wife immediately. "Pray for the dead. There will be many." I explained that I would stay to finish out the workday. I spent the rest of September 11 in the only governmental building in Washington that stayed open that day. The federal government workers could go home; the physicians could not. The sick still required tending.

The staff at the VA had been sent word that we might be needed at the nearby hospital in Arlington to help with the wounded from the Pentagon. As it turned out, there were few wounded. Most of those within range of the explosion had not survived. Sadly, we were not needed across the river at the other hospital.

After the terrorist attacks, we received government-mandated lectures on bioterrorism. A resident had treated one of the local cases of inhalation anthrax, so she gave a presentation on treatment of this disease. She stressed the importance of having a low "index of suspicion" for obtaining a chest X-ray in local patients, with the possibility of this disease lurking. There was a particular finding they had noticed on the chest film of the anthrax patient that later proved to be an early sign of the disease. Given the relative paucity of cases, not much was known about the diagnosis, so this was a potentially important discovery.

We also received lectures on smallpox, complete with information on the purported possibility of such a threat. We saw graphic pictures of this terrifying disease, which causes excruciating death in up to 30 percent of cases: the blistering skin lesions that burst, oozing fluid until the patient dies of dehydration and burn-like wounds. We were given information on the risks and benefits of the vaccine, which could potentially prevent, but was also known to sometimes cause, smallpox. In the event of an outbreak, as healthcare workers, we would be among the first to be vaccinated.

We were also told of the "treatment" once someone contracts smallpox: isolation and morphine for pain control. Most likely, lots of morphine. What they neglected to explain to us was the following: Smallpox could, and should, have long ago been entirely and definitively eradicated from planet earth. To do so was, and still is, entirely within the capability of humankind. The only smallpox viruses left are in bioweapons laboratories maintained by the United States and foreign nations. A collective and cooperative agreement to destroy these samples would forever put an end to the threat, but we have not done this.

"If they have it, we need to have it too," goes the morbid logic of bioweapons researchers. This research—often euphemistically relabeled as "biodefense" for public relations purposes—is a death cult. Covid should have taught us the folly of "gain-of-function" (that is, bioweapons) research, but we steadfastly refuse to learn. We instead busy ourselves trying to solve terrifying problems of our own creation.

A few months later, "The Sniper" struck Washington, DC. This psychopath lurked in the shadows. An expert marksman, he picked off unsuspecting pedestrians in parking lots with his long-range rifle. Primed by the threat of another terrorist attack, and endangered by a sharpshooter who seemed to enjoy putting bullets through the heads of random innocent victims, tensions in the city rose markedly. Some people refused to get out of their cars, while others refused even to leave their homes. It felt as though the threat of violent death was all around.

Having spent the past year working in hospitals, I was exposed to a sobering fact that we tend to forget or ignore in our everyday lives: Sniper or no sniper, terrorists or no terrorists, death can strike any of us at any time. Seeing it on the evening news, however, makes denial more difficult. Our psychological defenses weaken.

One year later, while on my surgery acting internship rotation, the intern and I were shooting the breeze. A dedicated, hardworking doctor, he was full of advice for me and frequently offered nuggets of counsel. He had just hung up the phone in disgust. Another physician had ordered a medication for the intern's patient that the patient was seriously allergic to—an allergy clearly documented in the chart.

Fortunately, the intern canceled the order before the drug was given. He was not happy about the incident.

"Just remember," he told me, "in the hospital, you are surrounded by assassins: There are incompetent people everywhere trying to kill your patient." That seemed a bit paranoid at the time. Now, I'm not so sure.

Terrorists, snipers, zebras. DC was deadly that year. The denial of death became for a time more difficult. Our defenses were down.

During an emergency medicine rotation later that year, a thirty-six-year-old woman came to the ER after a syncopal episode (the medical term for fainting) that had occurred while she was visiting her mother, who was also a patient in the same hospital. We began the workup, trying to figure out why she had fainted. But something was not so routine about this patient. After regaining consciousness, she had profound muscle weakness throughout her body. She could barely move her limbs, and was unable even to sit up. We thought little of this at first; however, after hours in the emergency room, her strength had still not returned. We continued to run tests to rule out other possible causes, to no avail.

After numerous trips in and out of the patient's room to re-examine her, I eventually picked up bits and pieces of the family's conversation and realized what had been happening around her when she fainted. The patient—at that point a visitor in the hospital—and her family were scheduled to meet with their mother's doctor that afternoon. The purpose of the meeting was to decide whether or not to discontinue their mother's intensive life support. The mother was on a ventilator, her prospects for recovery very poor.

I began to guess the source of the patient's muscle weakness. There was, in fact, nothing wrong with her brain, her nerves, or her muscles. The problem, I surmised, originated in her mind. I began to suspect that my patient was deathly afraid—not of death itself but of the responsibility for the end-of-life decision. She was having what psychiatrists call a "conversion reaction." Conversion disorders—what used to be called hysteria in the nineteenth century—are a heterogeneous group of psychiatric phenomena, all of which involve psychological conflicts manifesting as neurologic symptoms, often mimicking another disease. One can have conversion paralysis, conversion epilepsy (also called pseudo-seizures or non-epileptic seizures), and even conversion blindness.

Conversion disorders are a mental defense against severe psychological stress. They are a means of escape from an intolerable double bind. This reaction is not simply a matter of the patient "faking" a bodily symptom. A person with conversion epilepsy, for example, is not merely pretending, or consciously intending, to have a seizure.

I hypothesized that this patient's conversion reaction resulted from the fear of having to make a decision that might foreseeably hasten her mother's death. I learned that she was the primary decision-maker as her mother's legally designated healthcare agent. In a few hours, when the family met with the physicians, she would have to make the call; the burden ultimately rested on her shoulders. She did not want to abdicate this responsibility. She had to be, as she kept insisting to me, "the strong one."

The medical and legal system had unfairly framed the situation such that our patient felt responsible for her mother's death. What a terrible burden we placed on her! Our deployment of medical technology in the form of ICU care—the ventilator and all the rest—had created this situation, where such a decision needed to be made in the first place. And everyone was looking to her for the answer, which was more than she could (or should) bear. Our whole intensive biomedical approach to end-of-life care, not some disease her mother had contracted, was responsible for laying this intolerable burden on her shoulders. Her paralytic illness was iatrogenic—caused by the medical system itself.

Her conversion paresis provided a way out of her dilemma. As long as she was unable to walk, we insisted she stay in the ER. So it was not her fault that she could not make the decision. Although not conscious of this fact, she was, quite literally, paralyzed by fear.

I ran this hypothesis by the attending. He concurred, saying that he had also suspected a psychogenic origin, although he was unaware of her particular stressor.

I went back into the patient's room and sat down beside her. This time I did not ask her about her symptoms, or have her try to lift her legs, squeeze my fingers, or turn her head, as I had done before. Instead, I spoke to her of her moral dilemma.

"I understand you have a very difficult decision to make."

She nodded. "Yes." Then she looked at me.

"You have a lot of family members here. But ultimately, you have to make the decision about your mother's care. Is that correct?"

She nodded again, silently.

"That is a heavy burden to bear," I went on. "You do not have to do this alone: The doctors also want the best for your mother. They are there to help. Your family is here to support you. You are not alone in this. They will support you in whatever you decide."

The patient began to weep.

"I know you are afraid. I know you are worried that you might make a bad choice."

Her crying intensified. She wiped the tears from her face. *Movement of the arm—good.*

"You will make the right choice. Do not worry," I said slowly. "You will make the best decision, and your family will stand by you." In a sane and healthy society, death is a communal affair to be dealt with by the entire community. Traditional societies do not place decisions about death on the shoulders of one person, as we often do today. No one should have to face death—their own or a loved one—alone.

I asked the patient to sit up. Still crying, she did so.

"Now, I want you to try to stand."

She nodded in assent. Then, gingerly, as if to save face, she stood up. Her hand on her brother's arm, she then walked slowly out of the emergency room toward the elevator.

I don't know what she decided. But I do know that her illness, her temporary impairment, was our fault. Medicine foists burdens on families that we ourselves run from. We designate someone else to decide and wash our hands clean of the very burdens that our own technologies and techniques have created. In the medical ICU, we create a self-perpetuating system of intolerable decisional burdens that we lay on others without a willingness to shoulder them ourselves. "Here is your menu of medical options—take your pick . . ."

When further medical intervention is clearly not beneficial, the reasonable and merciful decision is to let the disease take its natural course, even when this means that death may be foreseeably hastened. This does not mean we aim at or intend the death of a fellow human being—as the shortcut of euthanasia does to our detriment. We doctors can forget, especially after death becomes routine on the wards, that in truth, death is dreadful. And the death of a loved one is anguishing. Even for those with the hope of heaven, dying is a mystery laced with trepidation. Death remains an enigma, the great unknown. We understandably resist, even rage, against its inevitability, as poet Dylan Thomas wrote in these bracing lines:

> *Do not go gentle into that good night,*
> *Old age should burn and rave at close of day;*
> *Rage, rage against the dying of the light.*[15]

It's natural to resist death. Perhaps there are circumstances in which we should rage against the dying of the light. But contemporary medicine risks only amplifying this rage. When medicine impedes our dying, but without actually providing life with new light, the burden falls on patients to learn on their own to go gently—often in spite of medical pressures pushing in the other direction. The burden also falls on family members to resist the momentum of our medical machinery and instead allow their loved ones to go gentle into that good night at the close of the day.

Saint Thomas Aquinas, clearly a believer in eternal life after death, examined the subject of death with the sober realism of one who knew himself to be a mere creature when he wrote that of all bodily evils, death is the most fearful: It is the most extreme of all human suffering, in which one is robbed of what is most lovable: life and being.[16] Despite all our therapeutic efforts to "cope" with death, there are no formulas or methods for contending with the final privation of life. The schema of Elisabeth Kübler-Ross's well-known stages of dying—denial, anger, bargaining, depression, and acceptance—tells us nothing about how to negotiate this hard road to acceptance, how to surrender in the end. It is perhaps a map of the terrain but not a guide through it.

In his provocatively titled 1974 article "The Indignity of 'Death with Dignity'," bioethicist Paul Ramsey suggests that "there is an additional insult besides death itself heaped upon the dying by our ordinary talk about 'death with dignity'."[17] Physician Sherwin Nuland, in his more macabre book *How We Die: Reflections on Life's Final Chapter*, argues along the same lines, writing that the concept of a "good death" is mostly an illusory wish.[18] Death is usually a messy, tragic, sorrowful business, accompanied by anguish and difficulty.

This is not to deny that some people experience a peaceful or painless death. On the contrary, many do die without fear and trembling. For many people today, this is the best we can hope for. We naturally want our death to be without suffering. While this wish is understandable, when this constitutes the beginning and end of a good death, it is also a sign of our diminished times. Escaping suffering at all costs was not always the highest priority for people preparing for death.

I am no stranger to pain and would be the last person to trivialize it. Following a ruptured disk and two failed spine surgeries, I experienced almost five years of daily, unremitting, debilitating, and incapacitating pain. On one occasion, the pain was so severe that I blacked out for twenty minutes. I spent the better part of those five years lying on my back. While it's impossible to quantify, I would wager that in one month during that period I experienced more pain than many people have endured in a lifetime. I would not wish a single day of this pain on my worst enemy. Every ounce of relief I got from medicine—including from the much-maligned opioid medications—I count a great blessing.

And yet, there are worse things than pain, and I would wager there are worse deaths than painful deaths.

Surprisingly few of our forebears prioritized a painless death above all else. A traditional Christian prayer pleads, instead, "From a sudden death, O Lord, deliver us." The worst kind of death was not a *painful* death, but a *sudden*, unprovided-for death that robbed one of the opportunity to adequately prepare. This traditional attitude suggests that death is not mere extinction of life, but a last duty laid upon us to perform—one that reveals the quality of our character.

There is more to death with dignity than an absence of suffering, and suffering itself does not rob a person of dignity. It is little wonder that those who believe this alone is necessary for a dignified death want to offer assisted suicide or euthanasia to those who do suffer at the end. A soldier who dies for his country: That's death with dignity. A martyr who dies for her faith: That's death with dignity. An old woman who dies after reconciling with her estranged daughter: That's death with dignity. By contrast, the absence of suffering alone doesn't equate to death with dignity. An AIDS patient who dies in agony can also die with dignity. I have seen it happen.

Yes, of course, we should treat pain at the end of life—and at every other stage of life. But our dignity comes not from a pain-free or unbloody end. It comes from reconciliation, from surrender, from acceptance. It comes from commending one's animating, life-giving principle—one's soul, to use an old-fashioned term that has not been improved upon—into the hands of Another. This is the opposite of suicide, for to kill is not to die, and to be killed is not to kill.

We did not ask to exist, but we have to make a go of it. This begins with a grateful acceptance of life. And, what is typically more difficult, a grateful acceptance of death when it comes. "Man is but a reed, the most feeble thing in nature; but he is a thinking reed," wrote the great scientist-philosopher Blaise Pascal. He continued, "The entire universe need not arm itself to crush him; a vapor, a drop of water suffices to kill him. But even if the universe were to crush him, man would still be nobler than that which kills him, *because he knows that he dies*, and the advantage which the universe has over him; the universe knows nothing of this" (emphasis added).[19]

Knowing that we will die frames our entire life. If we were destined to never die, if anything done once could be repeated endlessly, our actions and our relationships would lack ultimate significance. Feeble, finite, and mortal as we are, our knowledge of our own mortality paradoxically allows us to transcend our finite bodily existence. This transcendent element in us constitutes our true dignity. The only life we can "have" is a life that can be surrendered when our time comes—an act that only human beings, among all the animals, are capable of doing. The widespread use of extreme artificial life prolongation, now standard in medicine, means that death often involves succumbing rather than accepting, as German philosopher Robert Spaemann observed.[20] But we need not merely succumb. We can learn to surrender freely.

Medicine must likewise learn to yield modestly before this mystery of human mortality. For in the face of death, medicine finds itself out of its depth. Instead of trying to master death, medicine needs to acquire the ability to stand aside when the time comes. Whether we can learn to do so remains an open question.

CHAPTER 5

Heal with Steel

The wounded surgeon plies the steel
That questions the distempered part;
Beneath the bleeding hands we feel
The sharp compassion of the healer's art
Resolving the enigma of the fever chart.
             —T. S. Eliot, "East Coker"[1]

My job was to hold the leg. Until I was holding *just* the leg. The electric saw was buzzing, bits of bone were flying, and a tendril of smoke wafted up from the point where saw met bone. We were performing an amputation.

It was a surprisingly quick operation, no more than half an hour. Above the knee, the resident made a circumferential cut with a scalpel, tied off the few major leg vessels, and continued cutting until he reached bone. Then it was time to pick up the saw, an instrument that did its work quickly . . . until the leg came off in my hands, floating free from the patient's body. It was heavier than I expected. I handed it to a nurse, who put it in a plastic bag marked "biohazard" and carried it out of the operating room. I wondered what they did with these biohazards.

Surgeons traffic in body parts. They claim to heal with steel. Amputation was, admittedly, a strange way to heal. The operation was necessary, but no less bizarre for that. The leg was already useless to the patient: The vessels were so clogged that the foot no longer received adequate blood supply and had developed gangrenous ulcers. The patient had not walked on this leg for some time. Without amputation, the gangrene would eventually cause a deadly infection in his blood. The leg was already "dead," and death cannot live in symbiosis with life for long; it seeks the company of other body parts and eventually, of the entire body.

I had handled other detached body parts before, and not just cadaver parts in gross anatomy lab. I thought back to the liver. Unlike the amputated leg, the liver was not dead. The situation was reversed: The "living" body part had been removed from a dead body and kept artificially "alive" to be put back into a different living body whose liver was more or less "dead." A liver transplant—an astonishing feat.

I thought back also to the kidney, also a different situation. For that body part had not been removed from a dead body to be transferred to a living one. It had been removed from a living body and was itself very much alive. In this situation, the kidney was considered a "spare part," since its twin would remain inside the donor and take over the function of the donated body part. Taking living body parts from the living so that another may live—another astonishing feat.

Of all these body part removals and transfers on which I assisted, amputation seemed the worst. One does not notice a missing kidney—the body compensates, and unless the other kidney becomes diseased, life for the kidney donor goes on as before. But after losing a leg, everything changes.

Mr. Sowell was a forty-two-year-old double amputee, both above the knee. By contrast, a below-the-knee amputee retains some function. The patient can usually walk, since prosthetic legs work much better when the person has a functional knee joint. With above-the-knee amputations, especially when both legs are gone, one is confined to a wheelchair. This was Mr. Sowell's unfortunate situation.

He was not accustomed to spending time in a chair. He had worked the railroad, as his father had done, laying down tracks.

"My dad told me I wouldn't be able to do that job," he recounted. "Said I wasn't tough enough." And then, laughing to himself, he said, "I showed him."

After the railroad, he had worked construction, operating a tractor. His body showed signs of these years of hard physical labor: His muscular barrel chest, his thick beefy arms, his trim waist, and his bull neck attested to his former professional work. Mr. Sowell possessed a solid, salt-of-the-earth, working-class self-respect. He was proud of his professional accomplishments and proud of proving his father wrong. Mr. Sowell was indeed tough enough.

When I first saw him, his second leg had just been removed, less than a year after the first was taken. Otherwise healthy, severe vascular disease was his scourge. This disease apparently ran in his family, and his uncle was also a double amputee. While recovering from his second amputation, Mr. Sowell showed signs of depression. He wept frequently.

My final month in medical school, I was finishing my surgery AI on the vascular team. Mr. Sowell was one of my patients.

As a future psychiatrist, I was more interested in the psychological effects of surgery than the surgeries themselves. I took an interest in Mr. Sowell and spent extra time chatting with him. He spoke at length about his uncle. Because he was a teacher, Mr. Sowell's uncle could continue in his profession after he lost his legs. He was not supposed to drive, but he rigged devices in his car that allowed him to manipulate the pedals. The state patrol knew his situation and told him that they would leave him alone as long as they did not see him swerving around on the road or otherwise having difficulty. He continued to drive to work every day. When he arrived at school, his fifth-grade students would race out to his car to see who would be the first to get his wheelchair out of the back seat or the first to help him into it.

Mr. Sowell clearly admired his uncle's grit. Unlike his uncle, however, he could not go back to his old profession. He would have to start over. He had lost much more than just his legs.

Lying there in the hospital bed, he couldn't see any options. He began to despair. The life he had known, his role in the drama, was going to change drastically. Nothing in his prior experience prepared him to see the road ahead. But gradually, as the days went by and our discussions continued, Mr. Sowell's outlook began to shift. He talked more about going back to rehab and began thinking of other things he used to enjoy that he'd still be able to do.

Medicine took something from him—granted, it took his leg to preserve his life, a bargain that most of us would strike. But it offered little to help him contend with this loss. We amputate and leave the patient to deal with the aftermath. Some patients have supportive communities and networks to help them navigate these waters. But in our increasingly fragmented society, where loneliness has become an epidemic, many others do not.[2] His surgical wound would heal, but without community, healing the deeper wounds would be virtually impossible.

One of the most difficult things about being a medical student, I found, was being unable to follow up. After the patients were discharged, I typically never found out what happened to them. I do not know what became of good Mr. Sowell. I hope that he has found his niche, his new place in the world.

As my third-year transplant surgery month wound down, I had yet to see a liver transplant. I had assisted on a kidney donor surgery already, but the liver cases were few and far between.

Many students on the rotation never got the opportunity to see a liver transplant. The kidney operation had gone well, with only one minor glitch: The surgeon had dropped the detached kidney inside the donor's body. You wouldn't think this would be too problematic—just reach inside and pull it out. This operation, however, had no large incisions into which one could reach. It was done laparoscopically.

The patient had only four tiny incisions, three of them no more than a centimeter long, the other only a few centimeters—just wide enough to squeeze the kidney through for removal. Through two of the smaller incisions, the surgeon inserted surgical instruments. Through the other, she inserted the camera. The abdomen had been inflated with carbon dioxide gas so that the surgeon could see what was inside through the camera lens. We watched the operation on one of two television monitors in the room.

Using the two surgical instrument arms, the attending, Dr. Katz, placed the detached kidney into a small plastic bag for easier removal, and guided it toward the larger incision. Just as she got the body part to its exit point, the kidney slipped out of the instrument's grip and disappeared from view on the screen. The resident guiding the camera could not locate it. After detaching an organ from its blood supply, time is critical: It must be rapidly transferred to an ice bath so that the tissue does not die from lack of oxygen before it is placed into another body and blood flow restored. There was little time to waste. We had to locate the missing kidney and quickly remove it from the patient's abdominal cavity, or the precious body part would be of no use.

"Fuck! Fuck! Fuck!" shouted Dr. Katz—a habit of speech for which she was well-known. She yanked the surgical instruments from the small laparoscopic incisions. The open holes began to exhale carbon dioxide, as the patient's abdomen deflated.

"Put your finger here," she commanded, grabbing my hand. I plugged the two open holes with my index fingers and the belly stopped spewing hot air. Sometimes you must improvise in the operating room, and a medical student's two fingers were as good a plug as anything. I felt like the little Dutch boy with his fingers in the dam.

"Scalpel," she ordered. Taking the knife, she extended the larger incision a few more centimeters. She had tiny hands—the smallest surgeon hands I had ever seen—and was able to stick one hand through this slit. For a few tense seconds, she groped around blindly inside the patient.

Until finally: "Got it."

Well, that's not something you see every day. This was one of those minor complications the patient never hears about: no damage done, no reason to know. Losing the kidney for a few tense moments. Just a little bump in the road.

The difference with a liver, of course, is you only have one of them, so no living person has a spare to give away. One morning, prior to transplant rounds, I received some good news.

"Go ahead. You can tell the patient," the resident said.

Like so many others on the transplant service, Ms. Hahn had cirrhosis of the liver. Unlike the others, however, her disease was not caused by excessive alcohol consumption. She was born with a genetic disorder, alpha-1-antitrypsin deficiency. This disease involved the absence of a protein enzyme crucial for liver and lung function. The deficiency slowly destroyed her liver, until, in her fifties, Ms. Hahn had become seriously sick. It was at this point that we were taking care of her in the hospital while she awaited a replacement organ—the only thing that could save her life.

Transplant organs are distributed on an "as needed," rather than a "first come, first served," basis. After an extensive medical and psychiatric evaluation, a patient can be placed on a regional transplant list to wait for an organ among the other patients from nearby states. The more ill one becomes, the closer one moves toward death, the higher one moves up on the priority list. After arriving at the top of the list, the patient and doctors hope that an organ becomes available before the disease kills the patient. Ms. Hahn was now at the top of the regional list. She was getting sicker by the day.

I woke her from sleep. She looked at me, eyebrows raised, examining my expression.

"I have some good news for you, Ms. Hahn," I said. She leaned forward. "You're getting a liver today." A broad smile crept over her face. She squeezed my hand.

"Really?" she asked, almost in disbelief.

"Yes." I grinned back.

"Do I have time to call my brother?" she asked. "He wants to fly in from California."

"Sure. Your liver won't arrive here for a few hours. We'll take you to the operating room early this afternoon."

Just an hour before this, a young man had died suddenly in a motorcycle accident. While it sounds callous, sudden death is good for donated organs—it keeps them fresh. In one man's death was another woman's promise of life. It's uncomfortable to acknowledge, but in transplant medicine, "the living are parasitic upon the dead."[3] One of the transplant attendings, Dr. Smith, was en route from a nearby hospital to Georgetown, carrying a special delivery in an ice chest. On his way, he stopped at a fast-food joint.

"I was hungry," he later confessed during the surgery. "A cheeseburger sounded so good." The guy at the drive-thru window probably never would have guessed what the passenger was carrying in his trunk.

Before you can remove a liver for transplant, the patient must be declared "brain dead"—the current medical criteria for death, which involves the total cessation of all brain activity. Advocates for brain death criteria argue that death is the disintegration of the unified organism, and the brain is responsible for maintaining organismic unity. But this rationale does not actually stand up to scrutiny. The brain modulates the coordinated activity of the other organs, but it does not create this coordinated activity. That is accomplished by the organic formal unity of the body as a whole—which modern science, with its reductionistic analysis of the body into component parts, cannot see.

Although a brain-dead patient has no functional electrical activity of the brain, the patient continues, with the help of machines, to breathe and to circulate blood. The organs continue functioning, keeping them fresh for transplant. The body of the brain-dead person on a ventilator maintains homeostasis and coordinated unity of functions: The kidneys make urine; the liver makes bile; the immune system continues to fight off infections; wounds heal; hair and fingernails grow; endocrine organs secrete hormones; broken bones heal, and broken skin repairs; children grow proportionately as they age.

Pregnant mothers can even gestate babies after brain death, sometimes for months. Consider the inherent contradictions and manifest absurdities in this headline from the Associated Press: "*Brain-dead* Virginia woman *dies* after giving birth."[4]

To all appearances, a patient in this state does not, in fact, appear dead. This has led some medical ethicists—quite sensibly—to question the validity of "brain death" as an adequate criterion for death. For example, the prominent neurologist Alan Shewmon argues that "'Brain death as death' began as a utilitarian legislative decree and has remained a conclusion in search of a justification ever since: a conclusion clung to at all costs for the sake of the transplantation enterprise that quickly came to depend on it."[5]

The brain death criteria were developed by a Harvard Medical School committee in 1968 to free up ICU beds and promote organ transplantation—with death itself forming the foundation of the organ transplant enterprise. For organ transplantation rests upon a paradox—perhaps an outright contradiction—a "dead" donor whose body, with its precious organs, is still living.

After someone is pronounced brain dead, if the family refuses transplantation or if the organs are deemed unsuitable for transplant, the following situations emerge. Once the ventilator is turned off, the patient's heart may continue beating for several minutes, or even for a few hours (especially if the patient is a newborn). We would not send such a "dead" patient to the morgue, cremate her, or bury her while the heart still beats. Should we then give a drug, like potassium chloride, to stop the heart of the supposedly already-dead patient? In some cases, we wait a day or two to shut off the machines of the patient pronounced brain dead to allow family to travel from a distance to be at the bedside when the ventilator is discontinued and the heart subsequently stops. Is this family witnessing the death of the patient, or simply the cessation of efforts to animate an already-dead corpse? If the latter, why would family members want to be present for that?

Considering these oddities and absurdities that stem from the legal fiction that brain death is the death of the person, "total brain failure" is a more accurate term than "brain death." It indicates an irreversible coma, not a dead body. Perhaps such a person is "better off dead," as many people assume. Certainly, it is justifiable in such a situation, where meaningful recovery of human functioning is impossible, to discontinue life-extending measures such as ventilators or antibiotics. Even so, such a person is not yet dead. Total brain failure is a state where medical interventions should be discontinued because they cannot achieve meaningful ends. But it is likely not yet a state where the body's parts should be harvested at will.

The problem is, if critics of brain death are correct—and I find their critiques compelling and the responses to them unconvincing—this would spell the end of organ donation as it is currently practiced. But it would be many years after medical school that I began considering this matter in depth.

As a student, I was thrilled to scrub in on Ms. Hahn's liver transplant operation. It lasted twelve hours. First, her hardened, nodular, gray liver had to be dissected out, separated from its bile duct and blood supply, and removed. Like the amputated leg, this body part was carried away as another piece of biohazardous waste. Before we removed the liver, however, the largest vein in the body—the inferior vena cava (IVC)—which carries all the blood from below the chest back to the heart, had to be clamped. The liver wraps over the IVC, which runs behind it; the former cannot be removed without also taking the latter.

To accomplish this, the blood that normally flowed through the IVC was pumped through a hose that ran outside the patient's body, behind my back to a bypass machine, then back into her body and to her heart. Since this hose was much larger in volume than the IVC had been, the blood pressure would drop precipitously the moment we clamped the vein and the blood flow shifted to the hose. To counteract this effect, the anesthesiologist stood ready to administer rapid-acting medications that would raise the blood pressure at the precise moment when it otherwise would have plummeted to dangerously low levels. Each action, the clamping, bypassing, and medicating, had to occur in sync to allow continued blood perfusion to vital organs, especially the heart and brain. A mistake here could easily lead to a heart attack or stroke.

In Ms. Hahn's case, all these steps went smoothly. I breathed a sigh of relief.

With the liver out, time was short. Once the new liver was removed from the ice, it would have to be put into the abdomen, attached, and its blood supply restored quickly. This meant that the vessels that had been tied off for removal now had to be rapidly sewn back onto the new liver's vessels. The new IVC also had to be sewn to the old IVC stump on the posterior side of the fresh liver. Then, the bypass could be shut off, and blood flow could resume in normal fashion.

The doctors coordinated these actions in perfect sync, and this too went smoothly.

Before putting the new liver in, Dr. Smith called me over to a side table, where he was handling the life-saving body part. He turned it over in a bucket of ice, demonstrated its anatomy, and carefully dissected away any unnecessary surrounding tissue.

I placed my fingers in the cool ice bath and ran them over the organ's smooth surface. Compared to the knotted greyish-hard ugliness of Ms. Hahn's old liver, the new body part was a thing of beauty: browned from its large supply of blood, supple, and soft to the touch. Without a fresh supply of blood, it would not last long outside the ice bath.

Dr. Katz, who was still working with two other residents on the patient, preparing the empty space inside to receive its gift, called for the liver. Dr. Smith picked it up and carried it to the operating table. Carefully, he lowered the fresh body part into the patient's open abdomen. Then, both attendings went to work sewing the new cloth into the old. I watched in wonder. *What an extraordinary thing we are doing here.*

"Time for a break," Dr. Katz said after some time had elapsed. "Come on," she said, motioning to one of the residents and me.

There were still a few hours to go before the surgery would be finished, but the most difficult part was over. Dr. Smith and a second resident continued working, while the three of us "scrubbed out," removing our bloody gowns and gloves, and made our way to a nearby conference room. There we found cold Chinese food, left over from lunch that day, waiting for us. It was nearly midnight. Hungrily, we grabbed a plate and dug in. As I sat down, my stiff back and cramped legs thanked me. Nine hours standing is a long time to hold retractors and suction blood.

Although I had been working with her all month, I rarely conversed with Dr. Katz. She stood barely five feet tall, yet she was widely regarded as the most intimidating attending at Georgetown. I have already mentioned her propensity for profanity. From her sharp tongue, she frequently fired verbal arrows at the residents. Interns were terrified of her. Although she was much tougher on the residents than on the medical students, each of us secretly feared committing the unforgivable blunder that would bring her wrath down upon our heads.

Without warning, she struck up a conversation with me as we sat munching chow mein and kung pao chicken.

"What are you going into?" she asked.

"At this point, I'm leaning toward psychiatry. But I'm not sure yet," I said, hoping that she had in fact been addressing me.

"I almost went into psychiatry," she said.

"Really?" I could not picture it.

"Yeah. I loved it. Fascinating stuff. Only thing was, I couldn't stand all the group therapy garbage. Too much fluff, you know."

I duly nodded.

She continued, "Actually, surgery is a lot like psychiatry." I waited for the explanation, which was forthcoming. "We surgeons manipulate people's bodies, and you psychiatrists manipulate people's minds."

I suppose that's one way to look at it, I thought, but kept my thoughts to myself.

Ms. Hahn spent many days in the intensive care unit before awakening from sleep. The surgery had gone as well as it could have, but a liver transplant is so traumatic that her body needed several days of rest before she regained consciousness. When she finally awakened, her life had changed forever. For the rest of her days, she would take drugs that suppressed her immune system so that her body would not reject the foreign body part. This made her more susceptible to infections, but this was more than a fair trade for the benefits she had received.

She was no longer a patient with a terminal illness. She would live. And she lived because another was declared dead. Or mostly dead.

All transplant patients require a thorough psychiatric evaluation before placement on a transplant list. There are many reasons for this.

For example, a liver recipient may have destroyed his original liver by drug or alcohol abuse—hepatitis C from a dirty needle or alcoholic cirrhosis from excessive drinking. The psychiatrist must try to determine if a patient like this is likely to remain clean and sober after receiving a new liver. Such evaluations can be notoriously difficult. The psychiatrist has no crystal ball. His predictions are always, at best, an educated guess. The recipient must also be deemed psychologically stable and reliable enough to stay on the difficult regimen of immunosuppressant drugs after the transplant.

Living organ donors are also subject to psychiatric evaluation. Here, the psychiatrist must try to determine whether there is any coercion unduly influencing the donor's decision to give away an organ. In some countries such as China, there is a robust black market for donated organs, and poor people may be tempted to sell one of their kidneys. This rarely happens here, although there are other, more subtle forms of social coercion.

Such pressure can come even from well-meaning family or friends. "If you really loved your brother, you would do this to save his life," and so forth. People can feel trapped, as if they had no other choice than to undergo the knife for the sake of someone they love. Untangling the complexities of such situations is tricky, fascinating work.

As a fourth-year student, I observed the chairman of our psychiatry department evaluate a potential kidney donor. The man was a former cocaine addict. Now clean for eight years, he worked a steady job at a local bank. After kicking his drug habit, he had gotten his life on track. He loved his children; his marriage was stable. This man's brother was also a drug-addict, living on the street and dying of kidney failure. When he became sick enough, he showed up at the hospital for dialysis but otherwise stayed on the street. His family had offered him their homes and tried to help him get back on his feet, but he refused the aid.

The man we were evaluating described how one day, he was suddenly overwhelmed by this thought: He was supposed to give his brother one of his kidneys. He described this epiphany in religious terms.

"I don't care if he ruins the kidney I give him. I want to do it anyway," he insisted. Nothing we said could deter him.

"What if you knew that your brother would continue taking drugs?" asked the psychiatrist. "Would you still donate?"

"Yes. This is what I am supposed to do. I am supposed to help my brother, even if he doesn't want help."

While we found his sacrificial generosity admirable, the psychiatrist and I both worried that there was something unreasonable in his sudden impulse to offer unsolicited help that may not have been wanted.

"For all I know, his idea about donating a kidney may really be the result of a mystical experience," the psychiatrist later told me. "I don't really care either way. What concerns me is that nothing we say, no scenario we offered him, could deter him from this thought. There is something not quite right about it."

We finally made a bit of headway when we suggested that perhaps he was right.

"Maybe you are supposed to do something heroic to help your brother. But unconditionally offering him your kidney may not be the precise way you are supposed to help him. Perhaps you need to offer it on condition that he gets off the street and stays clean. This, after all, could be what really helps him."

It took some time, but he eventually came around. Help can take many forms, and the most important may not be high-tech, heroic medical interventions. As a recovered addict, this man did not want to become the ultimate enabler. If he could get clean, perhaps his brother could do the same. Tough love might be harder than giving away a kidney, but it's sometimes more effective. There are no easy fixes to a problem like addiction, no medical miracle cures. Medicine can assist, but the patient has to do the hard work.

"Can you tell us why you stopped taking your meds?" the psychiatry fellow asked.

The psychiatry fellow Adam and I were evaluating an eighteen-year-old man—or rather, boy, for he had a good deal more growing up yet to do—following a kidney transplant.

The surgery had gone well, his new organ had been in good working order for over a year, and he had enjoyed the freedom that came from being off dialysis—which, prior to the transplant, took up fifteen hours of his week. Then one day, he stopped taking his immunosuppressant medications. After a few weeks of this, his new kidney completely stopped making urine. Without his meds, his immune system rapidly destroyed the transplanted foreign organ. By the time we were consulted to evaluate him, the patient was in the hospital preparing to go back on dialysis. His new kidney was beyond salvaging. His negligence had ruined it.

During the initial interview, we spent almost two hours with him. We learned a great deal about him: his family life, social situation, work, and friends. He relayed his aspirations and goals, spoke of his childhood, and described his life with a chronic disease. After gathering sufficient background information, we began to probe for an answer to the question on everyone's mind. *Why had he stopped taking his meds?*

Yes, he knew what would happen if he did. No, he did not want to go back on dialysis. Yes, he was glad to have received the transplanted kidney. No, he did not simply forget about the medications. And so forth. There was no evidence of mental illness, yet he could give no justification for his action, could cite no influences, triggers, or purposes. After two hours, we were no closer to a rational answer.

Perhaps it was time to dig into the shadowy realm of the unconscious, where hidden motivations of self-sabotage might lurk? What might we discover there?

In good psychoanalytic fashion, we could posit any number of inner conflicts, defense mechanisms, or irrational motives. Proving any one of these would be nearly impossible, since the unconscious is, by definition, inaccessible to the patient. It was that much more inaccessible to us. The best we could do was guess, hypothesize, theorize. The patient's answer remained bafflingly consistent: "I don't know why."

Perhaps he did know but did not want to tell us. Or perhaps he was telling the truth: He was a mystery to himself, his actions as strange and inexplicable to him as they were to us.

On an unusually light rotation, Adam and I had been discussing the French existentialists.

"Have you ever read Camus's *The Stranger*?" I asked Adam. He had.

"You remember when the main character stood before the judge at the end of the book? The judge asked him why he killed that man on the beach. Remember his answer? 'The sun was bright. It was hot. I was sweaty and the sweat was dripping in my eyes and the sun was glaring off the water. So I shot him. I think I'll have another cigarette.' That was his defense, his reason for committing a totally inexplicable, senseless act. Well, that's our patient here. 'Why did you stop taking your meds?' 'I don't know. I was irritated. It was hot outside. So I stopped.' Or something to that effect."

Adam nodded in assent.

Camus presented his protagonist as a modern-day hero of sorts, a kind of postmodern saint who fearlessly faced the music of the world's absurdity. In truth, his protagonist was the absurdity.

Our patient sounded uncannily like Camus's protagonist, and this patient was anything but heroic. For no apparent reason, he chose to destroy a life-preserving, life-enhancing gift—a gift that could have gone to another patient who would have cared for it. He let the body part inside him die which had freed him from the chains of a dialysis machine. Now his life would once again be dependent on a sluggish, cumbersome, burdensome apparatus, with which he would live in uneasy symbiosis for many hours a week for the rest of his life. *Give him another kidney?* Perhaps someday. Perhaps not.

For now, however, the surgeons could think of only one thing to do for him. Consult the psychiatrist. This was a strange consultation, and the patient was the stranger.

"Morbidity and Mortality" conferences afford doctors the opportunity to learn from their mistakes. The weekly surgical M&M conference was a study in clashing egos. I enjoyed just sitting back and observing the action. Doctors present a case to colleagues in which there was some complication or suboptimal outcome. The other doctors scrutinize the details of treatment to discover what could have been done differently.

With surgeons, this sometimes resembled a courtroom drama. The "prosecuting" surgeons who were re-examining the work of their colleague had the benefit of hindsight and were often merciless in their examination. This, of course, made the "defendant" surgeon more defensive, though the ritual required that he not appear to be so.

The swaggering-surgeon stereotype stems from the necessary confidence that being a surgeon requires: It takes a certain kind of person to cut open another person. If he is not careful, the surgeon's confidence can inflate to unseemly proportions. A fellow medical student once characterized surgeons as follows: She stood erect and pounded her chest with both hands, all the while saying, "Aaahhh!" Then she paused, looked to the left and the right at those standing around her, and then resumed the chest pounding with an even louder, "AAAHHH!" She was playacting the physician as a chest-thumping gorilla—the alpha male asserting his dominance. This kind of power over life and death—the power to crack open the body and rummage around inside—tends to inflate the ego in some cases beyond what is healthy. It takes character to resist this pull—something that medical education today does not tend to cultivate.

During transplant rounds with Dr. Smith, we entered the room of a dying patient who had, among other medical problems, severe liver disease. Her family members were there. They were demanding that Dr. Smith do a liver transplant. He would not.

"As I explained before, her heart will not be able to handle the operation. The surgery would very likely kill her," he told them.

"She'll die anyway without the transplant," they replied. They had a point.

"I cannot do a transplant on her. It will kill her," he repeated, beginning to sound like a broken record.

"What are the odds she could survive the operation?" they insisted. "Give us a number."

"Less than ten percent."

"Well, that's better than her odds without the operation, which are zero. Ten percent is something. We're willing to take the chance."

Again, they had a point.

What Dr. Smith was thinking but did not want to say was this: The transplant team could not use a precious liver on a patient who would most likely die during the surgery. A liver is a rare resource. The recipient is therefore carefully screened and selected. Patients who could most benefit from this body part are given the gift. This patient's family, understandably, cared nothing about this problem of distributing a scarce resource. They knew only that their loved one was dying.

The conversation continued in much the same fashion for another ten minutes. Unable to convince the family, Dr. Smith extricated himself and made his exit. The rest of us filed out of the patient's room after him. After shutting the door behind him, Dr. Smith turned to me and asked with a heavy sigh, "Who says this job is easy?"

Nearly fifty years ago, one of the founders of American bioethics, Paul Ramsey, worried that some routinized and systematized approaches to organ transplantation could one day lead us to become "a nation of card-carrying precadavers."[6] When Ramsey coined this arresting phrase, the Uniform Anatomical Gift Act had recently passed, and every state had adopted this model legislation for organ donation. From our vantage point, half a century later, we no longer appreciate the radical novelty of organ transplant procedures—including the transplantation of paired organs from living donors.

But consider that never before in the history of medicine had we permanently injured perfectly healthy people in order to improve the health of others. Voluntary self-mutilation became, for the first time, permitted in law and practiced by medicine. With the advent of organ transplantation, we adopted new procedures that make a well person sick in order to make a sick person well—and we have not looked back since. We now regard this, quite rightly under some circumstances, as morally justified. Still, we should also regard it as extraordinarily odd.

Fifty years ago, the United States adopted an opt-in approach to organ donation after death. By contrast, the Netherlands recently joined Belgium and Spain in adopting an opt-out approach, with the default position that everyone is an organ donor upon death unless they specifically request otherwise. Similar legislation to switch to an opt-out approach was recently introduced in Britain and proposed in the US. This is not, I would suggest, a sign of moral progress. Voluntarily opting in seems more consonant with the integrity of man's bodily life and the logic of organ *donation*. In an opt-in system, organs remain always and only gifts to be freely given, not parts to be habitually taken.

Why is caution called for here? There is a real danger that we will increasingly view the human body as a collection of useful—or in some cases, not so useful—parts. The true self, as seen through our contemporary neo-gnostic sensibilities, is a kind of ghostly presence somehow inhabiting the mechanistic apparatus of the body. The philosophy of contemporary medicine—what the feminist writer Mary Harrington dubbed "meat lego Gnosticism"[7]—reinforces this view. The body becomes an assemblage of raw material whose components can be reconfigured or replaced according to the desires of the autonomous will. Or the almost-dead body becomes a repository of parts for harvesting according to the dictates of a managerial medical enterprise aimed at maximizing the number of organs procured from each opportunistic death.

In his book *The Anticipatory Corpse: Medicine, Power, and the Care of the Dying*, bioethicist Jeffrey Bishop advances the provocative thesis that modern technological medicine increasingly views the sick human body as though it were already dead. In modern medicine, the corpse is normative. Our philosophy of medicine imagines the living body only in terms of lifeless mechanistic causes, "the animation of dead matter," in Bishop's words.[8]

This is especially apparent in our care of the dying and in the ICU, where persons are often reduced to bare biological life, subsisting in a no-man's-land between life and death and sustained only by medical technology—from the ventilator that replaces the lungs to the dialysis machine that replaces the kidneys to the feeding tube that replaces the esophagus. "Dead anatomy begets physiology; physiology begets technology; technology—the replacing of a dead organ by a dead machine—begets a life worse than death," until eventually "the holistic care of the dying comes to look totalizing, indeed totalitarian," in Bishop's striking description.[9] The denizen of our ICU appears to be an animated corpse with tubes emerging from every bodily orifice.

But such an inhumane project to thwart death cannot be sustained forever. Repressed and banished, death seems to vanish from the horizon, but it crawls back in subterranean form. Modern medicine is continually struggling to master death, only to have death return with a vengeance. Death serves as the unconscious cultural and political motivator for medicine, indeed for much of contemporary society. As we explored in the previous chapter, our denial of death and our mechanistic philosophy of life have produced our totalizing medical system, blind to the lived reality of the human body and deaf to the full scope of a human life well lived.

We need a new medicine, attentive not just to decontextualized mechanistic forces—controlling blind biological functions without purpose—but attentive to meanings, intentions, loves, hopes, fears, and embodied purposes. That is to say, we need a medicine that treats human life as always embedded within a community and a context of meaning.

Consider that we always and only encounter our fellow human being in his or her corporeal, material life. A mechanistic or dualistic understanding of the human person undermines our capacity to care for one another precisely as bodily, sentient creatures. The generous gift of parts of ourselves in order to help another to live—the gift of organ donation—is always the action of persons of flesh and blood.

We are not merely interchangeable bodies, and our bodies are not just repositories of fungible parts.

While our system of organ donation in the United States attempts to maintain protections and restraints, dubious and dark international organ markets continue to spring up and grow like weeds. Although the Chinese government denies it, there is now compelling evidence that prisoners of conscience in China, such as members of the Falun Gong religion, are routinely killed and their organs harvested for profit.[10]

In the United States, thousands of desperate patients die every year waiting for organs that never materialize. To increase the number of available transplant organs, many today are pushing for an opt-out approach. Others are reviving proposals for the buying and selling of paired organs from live donors, or compensation for the next of kin of deceased organ and tissue donors. While motivated by laudable goals, these proposals are unwise, even if they would save lives.

Our system of organ donation should reflect the truth that our body is more than a commodity to be bought and sold. There are some things that money should not be able to buy.[11] Our body is not merely something we have. It is who we are. And there is a name for the sale of human bodies, which is slavery.

Perhaps an awareness of these truths about the human body, however dimly articulated, undergirded public indignation toward Simon Bramhall, a British transplant surgeon who pleaded guilty to charges of assault. The criminal charges came after it was revealed that Dr. Bramhall burned his initials onto the new livers of several transplant recipients during surgery. While the internal graffiti did not damage the liver or impair its functionality, the shock and blowback that this case triggered was severe and stern. The public understood that, however much this physician may have "worked" on these organs, they were not *his* work of art. As he submitted his resignation, Dr. Bramhall admitted, "It is a bit raw." To say the least.

The specter of a mechanistic dualism—in which the true self is a disembodied ghost in the machine, and the body is raw material for exploitation—continuously knocks at the door of modern medicine. In an age of efficient, turnstile medical machinery, where trafficking in body parts threatens to become routinized and industrialized, the organized *giving* of organs should be preferred to the routine *taking* of them.

When we consider donating all or part of our bodies, even for the noblest lifesaving purpose, it is imperative to maintain the logic of the gift. Generosity of this kind requires conscious and deliberate permission, with a full awareness of what is given and what is received. And we must attend more thoughtfully to the legal definition and medical assessment of death, for we should never knowingly kill one person even to save another.

What is more, the moment that trafficking in body parts ceases to seem strange, the moment we get used to this extraordinary exchange and come to see it as ordinary and mundane, something important for our humanity will be lost.

CHAPTER 6

Minds on Fire

All my joys to this are folly,
Naught so sweet as melancholy . . .
All my griefs to this are jolly,
Naught so damn'd as melancholy . . .
—Robert Burton, *The Anatomy of Melancholy*[1]

The patient lay motionless on the bed. I stood behind his head, holding an electrode probe in each hand. My mother stood at the foot of the bed watching me. When the doctor gave the order, I placed the two probes on either side of the patient's head, held them against his temples, and pressed a button. This caused electricity to pass through the patient's brain, inducing a generalized seizure, which lasted over one minute. "Well done, for your first time," the doctor congratulated me. My mom looked on, smiling. Was this some sort of bizarre nocturnal dream? Nope. Just another day in the life of a medical student.

I was administering ECT—electroconvulsive therapy. My mother was in town visiting. Since she worked as a mental health counselor and had treated clients who received ECT, she asked if she could accompany me to see how it was done. The attending agreed to let her observe the procedure. Psychiatrists sometimes still use this treatment for severe or refractory depression, manic-depression, catatonic states, and acute psychosis. The popular image of ECT for the layman is Jack Nicholson in the 1975 movie *One Flew Over the Cuckoo's Nest*, strapped to a table, flopping around and screaming, breaking teeth and bones. People also tend to think of ECT's predecessor—insulin shock therapy, as featured in the 2001 movie *A Beautiful Mind*. Both of these methods were indeed barbaric.

One of the chief reasons Georgetown's psychiatry department required all third-year students to observe ECT was to correct these misrepresentations. Things are done differently now. First, unlike Jack Nicholson, my patient lay perfectly still during his seizure, anesthetized, his muscles entirely relaxed. Second, save for exceptionally rare cases, ECT is no longer administered against a patient's will. When it is, careful legal measures are taken to ensure that it is done in the patient's best interest, and only when the patient is incapable of making rational decisions on his own because of mental illness.

Nevertheless, ECT remains controversial. Although it has fewer side effects than some psychiatric drugs and is even safe for both mother and baby in pregnancy, there is one adverse effect that mars the procedure. Some patients complain of persistent memory loss, usually of the events surrounding the procedure. The question arises: Does the treatment work because patients forget how depressed they were, or does it really treat the neurological cause of their depression, with the unfortunate side effect of memory loss? Perhaps it does both. In any case, if used judiciously, ECT can be a life-saving treatment. How does it work? There are various theories, but no one really knows. I think of it like hitting the reset button on one's brain, just as one would do on a computer when the software jammed up. But that's hardly a physiological explanation.

My first day of psychiatry rounds was eye-opening. The first patient entered the interview room and sat down. He was a flamboyant man in his mid-thirties, handsome and carefully groomed. "How are you this morning, Tom?" Dr. Chambers asked. Psychiatrists have the habit of addressing patients by their first name.

"Just fine," Tom answered. "I have been making plans. There is not much time left. You see, the moment is coming when the Sacred Triumvirate will bring order out of the chaos."

"The sacred triumvirate?" asked Dr. Chambers.

"Yes. I have to gather them together."

"Who are they?"

"Al Gore, Dick Cheney, and Colin Powell. They are destined to bring order out of the chaos."

"I see," said the doctor. "Tell us, Tom, why were you evicted from your apartment?"

"It was the neighbors below me. They hated me. They wanted to kill me. It was time to leave, anyway. I had to tell people about the Coming Times. I had to prepare them." For three days prior to his admission, Tom had been walking around the DC Mall, talking to anyone who would listen, explaining the coming of the sacred triumvirate and the need to bring order out of the chaos. After days of doing this, his shoes were worn thin. He had slept little.

"Why did your neighbors hate you and want to kill you?" asked Dr. Chambers.

"Because of the water." Tom explained that he had removed all plastic piping from the plumbing in his bathroom. This caused flooding in the apartment below him. "Plastic is not of the earth," Tom said. "It is part of the chaos. The wood and porcelain I left in place, because they are of the earth. It was necessary to do this, to bring order."

"I see," said Dr. Chambers. Tom had paranoid schizophrenia.

After we discussed the next steps to treat him, which involved adjusting his antipsychotic medication, treatment team rounds on psychiatry that day proceeded with a series of patients who were equally fascinating and beguiling.

The second patient, Julia, a slender, middle-aged woman, walked in and sat down. She glanced toward one side of the room then the other, got up out of her chair nervously, and began pacing the room, edgy and frantic. She spoke in a loud, pressured, anxious voice. Her words tumbled out with extraordinary rapidity, yet her mouth was still struggling to keep pace with her racing thoughts. "Bad vibes. Bad vibes from over there," she said, pointing to one side of the room, still pacing nervously. "It's a spiritual thing. I can feel it. Bad vibes."

"Hello, Julia. My name is Dr. Chambers." Julia had been admitted the night before with a diagnosis of acute mania. Dr. Chambers extended his hand, and she shook it. With the subtle touch of an experienced psychiatrist, he held her hand there for a few moments after the handshake, staring into her eyes with a calm smile. The gesture worked.

"Oh . . . good vibes. Good vibes from you," Julia said, releasing his hand. Julia was experiencing her first manic episode; we diagnosed her with bipolar disorder.

The next patient refused to come into the interview room. She had not left her bed for many days, except under duress. We walked into her room. The lights were out, and she became angry when we turned them on. "Leave me alone," she ordered.

"Nancy, can we talk with you this morning?" Dr. Chambers inquired.

"No. Let me die." Nancy had been discovered in her apartment by a neighbor, wasting away with severe clinical depression. She was found covered in her own feces, dehydrated and malnourished, the room in shambles. She refused medications. We were in the process of trying to get legal conservator status for her next of kin, so that he could make the decision for ECT treatment even though she objected. In the meantime, she stayed in her room, asking to die.

Rounds continued in this fashion with the rest of the patients on the ward. I was hooked.

One of my first patients on psychiatry was a man terrified of himself. Of all the tragic cases I saw during medical school, his was among the worst. Mr. Zimmer experienced intense auditory hallucinations commanding him to harm others, and intense visual hallucinations where he foresaw the results of the violent acts that the voices were ordering. For example, he described seeing a policeman on the street, and the voices commanding him to grab the officer's gun and shoot him. Then he looked at the officer and saw his chest blown open. Once, when he was cutting vegetables in the kitchen, the voices told him to cut the throat of his seven-year-old son. Mr. Zimmer was afraid of himself, terrified of what he might unwittingly do.

For a time, to get away from other people, he camped out in the mountains. But inevitably, he would see some hikers walking along the trail, and the voices would tell him to drive tent stakes through their heads. Mr. Zimmer looked the part of a violent man. He stood six feet tall, head shaved, muscular arms tattooed, wearing heavy black boots and a tank top. I was more than a bit nervous when it came time to draw blood on him, but he always greeted me cordially. He spent most of his time alone in a room, reading Fyodor Dostoevsky's *Crime and Punishment*, which seemed fitting, since the novel is a subtle psychological study of a man who murders someone. Mr. Zimmer was on close observation, with "sharps restriction," and thus, not allowed to eat with even a plastic knife and fork.

After several days on the ward with good behavior, Mr. Zimmer requested a walking pass, a privilege to stroll around campus with a staff member. We agreed, and I scheduled a time the next day to walk with him. When I arrived the next morning, the nurse pulled me aside. "Mr. Zimmer wants to kill you," she informed me. "He told me last night." I rescinded the walking pass.

The records from his prior hospital admission came via fax the next day. The reason for that previous admission was that he wanted to kill his doctor from his last hospital stay. In the past years, he had nearly thirty hospitalizations in at least three states. Doctors had met with little success in treating him. We did not fare much better.

A year later, I found myself sitting on a bench outside a courtroom. A small, elderly, pleasant-looking man came and sat beside me. "Is this where Judge Kirk's court is today?" he asked me.

"Yes. I think this is the right room. In fact, I'm waiting for him too," I told him.

"I'm James Jordan," he said, extending his hand.

"Pleased to meet you, Mr. Jordan" I said, shaking his hand, but not offering my name. I had suspected his name already, although his genial appearance caught me off guard. The night before, I had read Mr. Jordan's dossier. He had a hearing that day to request unconditional release and the right to live independently in the community. I was there to observe, as part of a forensic psychiatry experience.

That hand I shook had committed heinous acts. Thirty years ago, Mr. Jordan had shot his wife dead and attacked three of his children with a hammer. Two of his children, including the three-year-old, sustained serious head injuries. His mad rampage was triggered by the delusional belief that his wife had been unfaithful to him; he claimed also that he had been responding to voices commanding him to kill her. He pled not guilty by reason of insanity. His was one of the rare cases where this plea was successful. Contrary to popular belief, however, those who get off on a defense of insanity are not released back into the community.

He spent years in St. Elizabeths Hospital, a maximum-security mental hospital, where John Hinckley Jr., the man who shot President Ronald Reagan, resided until 2022. After his release from St. E's, Mr. Jordan had been living for years under close scrutiny of the court, which monitored his housing situation, his medications, mental health treatments, and substance abuse rehabilitation. This hearing was to see whether he could be released from the court's supervision.

The defense lawyer made a reasonably convincing case that Mr. Jordan was no longer a danger to others. The prosecution said very little, letting the historical facts of the case speak for themselves. Future dangerousness is notoriously difficult to predict. Studies show that housewives from Peoria do as well predicting future dangerousness as do clinical psychologists and psychiatrists. The only proven reliable predictive factor is a history of dangerousness in the past. Mr. Jordan lost the hearing. Whether this was just or not, I have to admit that I was relieved.

From these last two anecdotes, one might form the opinion that mentally ill people are violent by nature. This is not true; these cases represent exceptions to the general rule. When they are violent, the violence is almost always directed toward themselves, in the form of self-mutilation or suicide. The rare cases where a "crazy" person attacks someone else typically draw excessive publicity and media attention, thus skewing the view of the lay public and misrepresenting the situation of the mentally ill. These patients are much more likely to be the victims of violence than the perpetrators. Their mental illness may be the result of years of physical or sexual abuse, the horrors of war, or other tragedies.

Consider, for example, the case of a police officer I interviewed. This man suffered severe post-traumatic stress disorder, resulting from witnessing too many horrifying scenes on the job. The patient had lost his best friend while on duty, also an officer, who was shot dead at point blank range without provocation. The patient himself had shot and killed a man who was trying to kill him with a machete. Death threats from the victim's gang followed. He was the first to arrive on the scene of a murdered undercover officer; the man died in his arms. Shortly thereafter, he was the first on the scene of a nightmarish domestic violence incident involving an intoxicated father and his toddler son. So gruesome were the details of this last incident that they are not fit to print, although this did not stop the national press from doing so. Simply hearing it described by the officer disturbed me for days.

All these events happened within the span of a year. By the time the officer saw us, he was in bad shape. Like others suffering from mental illness, this patient, through no fault of his own and subject to forces outside his control, desperately needed help. There are countless stories like his from patients in veterans' hospitals, mentally marred from experiences of war. Then there are the children and teenagers whose stories of abuse or neglect seem almost unbearable.

I also witnessed baffling instances of self-inflicted pain that defied explanation. One night, while I was on my emergency medicine rotation, a man came into the emergency room after swallowing a razor. "Do you think he's telling the truth?" the emergency physician asked me after I presented the history.

"I think so," I replied.

"How should we find out?" he asked.

"The razor will show up on abdominal X-ray."

"Correct."

We looked at the X-ray. Sure enough, there it was. The razor had passed out of his stomach and into the small intestine. "Go ahead and page surgery," he said. The X-ray confirmed what I had suspected: The man had not lied. He claimed a prior history of swallowing a razor, which also had to be removed surgically. There was a corresponding large incisional scar on his belly. This could have been from any abdominal surgery, but he had another telltale sign that corroborated his story. He reported that years ago he poured gasoline on himself and lit himself on fire. Burn scars were strewn over his torso and legs.

"Why did you swallow a razor?" Here was a question I never imagined I would ask someone.

"I just wanted it to tear me up inside," the patient responded. Sadly, he got what he wanted: Before being taken to surgery, he began vomiting blood. The razor was indeed tearing him up inside. No doubt, something else, something hidden, was also tearing him up inside—tearing him up even before his deed of self-hatred made this metaphor a reality. What that something else was, I never found out.

Besides bearing the burden of their illness, the mentally ill bear the unjust social stigma of being "crazy," "nuts," or "weak"—unable to control their thoughts or moods, and somehow to blame for their condition. Like misperceptions of the mentally ill as violent, the idea that the mentally ill person is at fault is also false. People suffering clinical depression are often admonished to "snap out" of it, to pull themselves up by their bootstraps, as though their illness were self-inflicted or the result of some moral or spiritual weakness. But the great spiritual masters recognized the scourge of melancholy and knew that it could strike even those who do everything right. The ancient Christian desert fathers, for example, recognized the entity we now call clinical depression. They dubbed it the "noonday demon" and knew that it could afflict both novices that came to them seeking spiritual direction as well as the holiest and most seasoned monk. Mental illness can affect anyone. This makes it all the more frightening, all the more pitiable, all the more tragic.

How can we better help those with mental illness? Medicine alone cannot achieve this. Rates of schizophrenia do not appear to vary from one country to the next. While the research on this is still debated, several cross-national studies from the World Health Organization in the 1960s suggested that patients with schizophrenia in developing countries paradoxically have better outcomes—with fewer symptoms and improved social functioning—than those in developed and highly industrialized nations.[2] Given that the latter should have access to more advanced medical care, this finding continues to puzzle researchers.

Evidence suggests that antipsychotic medications and expensive psychiatric hospitals are not the most important prognostic factors for these patients. A supportive community where people are integrated, including strong extended family networks of support, may be more important for mental health than typical psychiatric interventions. Mentally ill individuals in underdeveloped countries may face fewer hostile remarks, find more opportunities for ad hoc work for those with disabilities, and maintain better social inclusion. The cultural context in which illness is experienced, and not just the availability of biological interventions, matters.

Those with mental illness often suffer in silence, hidden and unrecognized by others. A person with a medical diagnosis such as cancer will usually receive an outpouring of sympathy and support from their family and community; a person diagnosed with a mental illness, by contrast, frequently experiences isolation and inadequate support, often because of the unfair social stigma.

During the deinstitutionalization movement of the 1970s and 1980s, we emptied out the state mental hospitals. The old asylum system had its problems and abuses, to be sure, but the deinstitutionalization cure turned out to be, for many patients, worse than the disease. The pretense for closing the state mental hospitals was that the new antipsychotic medications would allow institutionalized patients to be treated successfully in the community. While these medications worked well for some patients, they were not the broad panacea that was promised. Many of those released languished in substandard conditions with inadequate help.

As a consequence, today our jails and prisons—indeed, our city streets—are filled with individuals who suffer from untreated severe and persistent mental illness. Prisons have become the nation's largest mental healthcare facilities: Between 10 and 25 percent of individuals who are incarcerated today have a serious mental illness, compared to 5 percent of the general population.[3] At least one-third of homeless persons struggle with serious mental disorders.[4] A decent society should not continue to accept this status quo.

To address the problem, we need to acknowledge that some patients may require prolonged civil commitment, as in days past, with appropriate legal due process and adequate safeguards to protect patients' rights. Letting these patients go untreated and abandoning them to languish on the streets hardly constitutes a respect for their rights, when their illness so impairs their mental capacity that they cannot make rational decisions or care for their most basic needs. More than institutional reforms, we need to become a society that refuses to regard those with severe and persistent mental illness as though they were invisible or less than fully human.

The patient stood by the window, looking out onto Georgetown's campus below. Light from the sun reflected off the windows of nearby buildings. People milled about on the sidewalks. Cars drove in and out of the parking lot. The trees were dropping their leaves.

"Do you see it?" the patient asked me, still looking out.

"See what, David?"

"The fire. That building there. It's on fire. See, the flames are leaping up."

"No, I'm sorry," I said, looking at him. A twinge of sadness came over me. I felt sorrow for him, for his wretched condition, for his standing there in a hospital gown on a locked psychiatric unit, looking out the window at the dazzling world outside, a world of sane people moving about freely.

"No, I am sorry, David. I do not see the fire."

CHAPTER 7

Only the Trying

Canst thou not minister to a mind diseased, pluck from the memory a rooted sorrow, raze out the written troubles of the brain, and with some sweet oblivious antidote cleanse the stuffed bosom of that perilous stuff which weighs upon her heart?
—William Shakespeare, *Macbeth*[1]

"Which patient would you like to see?" Dr. Burke, the psychiatry resident, asked me. "We have two down here: You pick one and I'll take the other. Room seven is a woman with bipolar, room nine a woman with depression. Both may be suicidal." We were standing in the emergency room, beginning our night on call.

"I'll take the patient with bipolar," I said. After glancing at the triage note, I walked into the room. The patient, a twenty-two-year-old student, sat slouched on the examining table. When I opened the door, she looked up, wiping tears from her face. "Hello," I said, sitting down. I introduced myself. She nodded.

I began questioning Lisa, plowing through the thirteen-page history and physical form we utilized to evaluate new psychiatric patients. Psychiatrists ask a lot of questions. I began with the history of her present illness, the events leading up to her coming to the hospital. Then, with this stranger who had never before met me, I bored more deeply into personal history, social and family history, drug history, sexual history. She offered the information freely, until we came to her history of suicide attempts. Here, she hesitated.

"Have you ever attempted to harm yourself?" I asked.

She looked down, pausing. "Yes . . . once."

"What did you do?" She hesitated again and looked away. "It's okay," I said. "You do not need to talk about it, if you are not comfortable." I moved on to the next subject. When I finished the interview and physical exam, I informed her that she might need to be admitted to the hospital.

She looked afraid.

"I need to talk with the resident first," I explained. "He'll come in here to speak with you as well. We'll make the decision after that. Have you ever been admitted to the hospital for psychiatric reasons before?"

"No," she said, almost inaudibly. Tears began to well up again. Her eyes pleaded with me.

"I will be back in a few minutes. Do you need anything?"

She shook her head. "I'll be okay."

I presented the case to the resident. The patient, Lisa, had been diagnosed with bipolar disorder—also known as manic-depression—a few years ago. She had a history of some manic episodes but suffered more frequently from depression. Her current melancholy was severe, although she was not presently contemplating suicide. In her words, she had gone to the brink but no further. Potential for self-harm or danger to others were the chief reasons for psychiatric hospital admissions, but Lisa could be admitted on the premise that she had failed outpatient treatment. Lisa later wrote in her journal, with obvious frustration, "How does one fail outpatient therapy? When one already feels like a failure, failing outpatient therapy is probably the most degrading experience one can have. Even if one tried very diligently to pass outpatient therapy." Her psychiatrist had recommended she come to the hospital that night.

Dr. Burke went into the room to question her. In five minutes, he learned more about the circumstances and reasons for her depression than I had learned in a twenty-minute interview. This came from experience. He was the finest resident I worked with during medical school and seemed to know just the right questions to ask. Later, when I asked him how he gleaned so much from the short interview, he pointed out that, unlike me, he did not have to plow through thirteen pages of required information, which helped him get to the heart of the matter.

"Dr. Burke agrees," I told Lisa. "We are recommending that you come into the hospital tonight. You will be safe here. I think we can help you." She did not appear convinced. "The psych ward here is not a bad place," I said, stretching the truth a bit. "It would be a good idea to call your parents." She nodded.

Her mother and father drove down from Delaware that night. When they arrived in the ER, the resident and I explained to them why their daughter could benefit from a hospital admission. They agreed.

Manic depression is a disease that interrupts a young person's life—usually beginning in their late teens or early twenties—without warning, and it is typically chronic and unremitting. It descends like a tornado, overturning years of life's work and plans, often leaving destruction in its wake. The disease involves biological factors, such as dysregulation of the brain regions responsible for "affective states" of mood and mental energy, but it is also influenced by psychological and social factors, such as adverse life events and stressors. Its hallmark is mania, a chaotic state of mind where the person can experience racing thoughts, grandiose delusions, pressured speech, extraordinary physical and mental energy, extreme agitation, and loss of sound judgment. When in a manic state, patients can go days on only a few hours of sleep yet not feel fatigued. Manic patients are typically euphoric, full of chaotic energy, though when they get too revved up, the euphoria can turn to irritability and agitation. They frequently get in trouble with the law, or spend all their money on foolish projects, since their capacity for rational thought is so impaired. The manic states last a week or more and are typically followed by a plummet into severe depression. Here, suicide is common. Half of all bipolar patients attempt suicide; one in six tragically will complete suicide.

During my first year of medical school, I learned that a close friend from high school had been diagnosed with bipolar disorder. A bright student who was talented in sports, Matt had gone on to a prestigious military academy where he was a varsity athlete. Shortly before graduation, his mental illness manifested. Symptoms began with mood instability, difficulty concentrating, and poor judgment. He became something of a class clown, even making wisecracks toward military superiors in front of others.

Despite this, Matt somehow managed to get his degree from the Academy. He continued post-graduate training for a career as a pilot, something that he had talked about since our high school days. This did not last. As his manic-depressive illness became progressively worse, he decided to self-eliminate from pilot training, a decision that haunted him for years afterward. He was given a medical discharge from the military. "Our pilots do not have bipolar," they informed him. After returning to his hometown, his professional dreams were shattered, and his erratic moods made it difficult for him to hold down a job.

This patient, Lisa, reminded me of Matt. Both were young, talented, successful students. Both had their lives interrupted by the same illness. I wanted to help them both, but there seemed to be little that I could do for either. I suppose Sigmund Freud would have characterized this as an instance of "counter-transference," where the therapist transfers feelings associated with a person or experience in his life onto a patient. Many films with psychiatric subjects build their drama around the phenomena of counter-transference—what the troubled psychiatrist himself learns from the troubled patient.

The day after we admitted her, I found Lisa sitting on the hallway floor of Five-West, the psychiatric ward, reading a book. She greeted me, relieved to see a familiar face. "What are you reading?" I enquired.

"T. S. Eliot."

"I hope it's not *The Waste Land*," I said. "That will probably make you more depressed."

"No, it's not," she said, smiling. "It's one of his shorter poems." But she may have thought, isn't this the wasteland? In the isolation room across from Lisa, a poor soul was belting out "Silent Night." Who knows what he was trying to silence.

"Eliot has a great line in the *Four Quartets*," I told her. "You should consider it while you are here, trying to make the best of the situation."

"What's that?" she asked.

"'For us there is only the trying. The rest is not our business,'"[2] I recited.

"Very good," she replied. "I'll remember that."

A night on the psych ward had not done much to lift Lisa's spirits. "It's so bleak up here. They could use some paint on the walls. Maybe some pictures," she said. I tried to explain that psychotic patients needed to minimize sensory inputs, which can provide fodder for their hallucinations. I did not mention that with suicidal patients on the wards, pictures were also out: Glass and metal frames could be used to cut. But I could not help agreeing with Lisa that the place could use some paint, maybe a bit more color.

Lisa was silent during group therapy. She did not like opening up in front of strangers. I did not blame her. "I never imagined I'd end up here," she told me. "I'd rather be in Paris. Have you ever been there?"

"I have. You won't be here long," I said. "I'd rather be in Paris, too." Later, from the stereo in the community room, I heard the Dave Matthews Band playing "Grey Street."

She thinks, hey—
How did I come to this?
I dreamed myself a thousand times around the world
But I can't get out of this place.[3]

"How is your mood this morning?" I asked.

"About the same. Pretty low. Not as bad as last night, though."

"Have you had thoughts of harming yourself?"

"No."

I presented Lisa's history on rounds that morning to the rest of the team. Then we interviewed her. She was a bright college student now living in a dark world. She had worked one summer for a former English teacher who was elderly and blind. Lisa would come to the old woman's house and read to her the stories of Geoffrey Chaucer's pilgrims. Now she was making her own arduous pilgrimage, traveling through a wasteland, her own mental state a blinding darkness.

We decided to stop her medication and switch her to lithium. We ordered the routine lab tests to check her kidney and thyroid function because lithium could adversely affect these organs. She reluctantly agreed to try the new drug. First, however, she made me photocopy all the pages that discussed lithium in a huge psychiatric textbook. She wanted to do her homework. To my surprise, she read them all. "You now know more about lithium than I do," I told her.

"I grew up Catholic," Lisa told me the next day. "I used to think about going off with Mother Teresa's nuns and working with the poor. Or maybe I'd go to a convent in Italy or something. I drifted away from the Church, but I still think about becoming a nun."

A lapsed Catholic who still wants to become a nun. You never know what you'll see next on psychiatry, I thought.

I had to draw blood from Lisa to send for the lab tests. "I'm not going to lie to you. This might hurt a bit," I said.

"Go ahead," she replied. I got it on the first stick, relieved to see the bright red fluid seeping into the vial. I sent the blood for testing.

We discussed her plans for finishing the semester. I suggested that she contact her school dean to get extensions on her finals, which were fast approaching as she sat in the hospital. "Maybe when you finish, you can go to Italy," I said. "Or Paris."

"I can't stand it here. I feel like I don't belong," she told me.

"I know. I realize it doesn't seem like it, but this is a good place for you right now." I replied. "You are safe here, and you'll be going home soon."

Yes, the psych ward is safe, Lisa thought. It is safe and suffocating.

The lab tests came back. Her kidney function tests were a bit off, but I suspected this was due to mild dehydration. She hardly drank anything. We stopped the lithium anyway. "You need to make sure you drink more water today," I said, giving her a bottle. "At least four of these. Just keep sipping on it."

"I never drink that much."

"Try. We'll run the kidney tests again tomorrow. Hopefully you can go back on the lithium." I was disappointed with this setback, having spent considerable time and energy trying to convince her to try the medication. She had even tolerated the first two doses well, which some patients did not. She was not pleased, either, still sitting as she was on the psych ward, which she had started calling "Grey Street."

A few months prior to my encounter with Lisa, I had visited my parents for a holiday, and Matt had stopped by to say hello. My eyes were immediately drawn to his neck. I did not have to ask what happened. I knew. On either side was a symmetric pair of three-inch horizontal scars. After a few minutes of conversation, I broached the subject, gesturing to his neck.

"Knife," he said, running his index finger over both scars. "Landed me in the hospital for a week. Very bad."

I could not get my mind around it. The gregarious kid of my high school days, who loved life and running and fishing and joking, had taken a knife to his throat. He had wanted to bleed out and end it. This knowledge crushed me. The Matt I had known from high school was the last person I would have expected to opt out of life, to turn in his ticket. But such is the havoc wrought on one's personality by manic-depressive illness. Matt's natural temperament, prior to his illness, was one of tireless tenacity combined with easygoing joviality. He loved joking around and was always the first to laugh at jokes we played on him.

Once in high school, we were on a ten-day backpacking trip in the mountains of British Columbia with seven other buddies and two guides. On day six, we decided that Matt, with his indomitable endurance, was hiking too fast for the rest of us. Despite the already heavy pack on his deceptively wiry frame, we could not keep pace with him. So we played a bit of a cruel joke on him by secretly burying twenty pounds of rocks in his backpack. Matt hiked all day, oblivious to the extra weight. When we stopped to make camp, he opened his pack and yelped out a Homer Simpson-esque, "D'oh!" He immediately suspected the prime culprit and yelled, "Kheriaty!" For a brief moment, I regretted the prank. But Matt's easygoing temperament got the best of his initial irritation, and he was the first to start laughing at the folly. Because of his good-natured reaction, we did not feel so bad laughing with him. He was always an easy guy to laugh with.

Matt made not one, but three suicide attempts. Each time, he changed his mind, interrupting the attempt before it proved fatal—sometimes escaping death only by a hair's breadth. Despite the ravages of his illness, which drove him toward self-destruction, he demonstrated an incredible will to live.

The first attempt occurred after experimenting with marijuana for the first and only time at a party one night. After smoking, his thoughts of suicide, undisclosed to anyone else, returned with a vengeance. After three straight days of constant self-condemning thoughts, Matt could not stand the mental torture any longer. He emptied an old bottle of pills into his hand, swallowed a handful, put on his scuba gear, and jumped into the lake behind his house. He sank to the bottom fifteen feet down and lay face up. The frigid January water seeped into his wetsuit and chilled his bones. Matt watched as bubbles from his respirator cascaded to the surface above. He could feel his heart beat more rapidly in his chest as his vision faded slowly in and out of focus. After an hour and a quarter, his wetsuit no longer adequately heating his body, Matt's teeth began to chatter against the oxygen regulator in his mouth.

He changed his mind. Matt inflated his equipment, floated to the surface, swam ashore, and painfully crawled up onto the beach in his backyard. After removing his mask and regulator, he doubled over with abdominal cramps, vomiting partially digested pills into a nearby hedge. Too weak to remove his wetsuit, he crawled into bed with it on for the worst night's sleep of his life. Initially, he awoke every few minutes to vomit the remaining contents of his stomach. After an hour of this, his stomach was empty, but the dry heaves continued, burning his throat with gastric acid.

When he awoke the next morning, Matt vowed never to experiment with drugs again. He attributed his suicide attempt solely to the effects of marijuana rather than his manic-depressive illness. He naïvely assumed that his mental state would spontaneously normalize if he stayed clean and sober.

The next fall, Matt enrolled in community college and began taking courses in instrumentation, but his mood remained irritable and his thinking erratic. When one of his teachers asked for written feedback from the students, Matt described the teacher as a "tinhorn dictator who turns a seemingly placid environment into a quagmire of human indignance and tyrannical domination." The teacher found this critique quite humorous, and for some reason this endeared Matt to him. Not everyone found Matt's increasing irascibility so funny, least of all Matt. During this time, his self-critical thoughts returned, and the incessant negative mental chatter increased.

I suspect every suicide attempt, however determined the suicidal person appears, is accompanied by some degree of ambivalence. Poet Robert Lowell wrote, "A doubtful suicide should choose the ocean / Who knows, he might reach the other side?"[4] For his second attempt, Matt chose not the ocean, as Lowell recommended, but the same lake as his first attempt. Although rationality told him he could not, perhaps Matt unconsciously knew that he could reach the other side. This time, he hiked out with his dog to a trail at the end of the road, stripped stark naked, said goodbye to the dog, and dove in. The March water was still frigid from the winter, surely too cold for him to last long. He began to swim, assuming that hypothermia would overtake him somewhere in the middle of the lake.

It did not. With relentless determination, he somehow managed to reach the other side. Beyond exhausted, Matt once again crawled onto the beach, blue and shivering, this time at the house of a stranger. The bewildered but hospitable residents took the naked young man in. While Matt emptied their hot water tank with a long shower, the kind strangers called his mother who came to get him.

Even after this attempt, Matt refused to resume psychiatric treatment. He could not accept his mental illness, could not see that bipolar disorder was the driving force behind his tormented thoughts and black melancholy. It took a third and more nearly deadly suicide attempt for him to accept this. This time, he headed out on another trail, not to a lake, but toward the mountains. He was alone.

Earlier that day, while sitting in class, Matt thought to himself, "This will all be over by this afternoon." He slipped out of class early and purchased a bottle of whiskey, a can of paint thinner, and a razor blade. Then he drove immediately to a remote hiking spot, a place familiar to him. A mile or so up the trail, he stopped hiking and knelt beside the river.

Normally an avid outdoorsman, Matt saw this as a final act of defiance. Anger churned inside him. He could not take any more mental torment—the racing, irrational, confused thoughts; the endless mental anguish; the critical voice inside that constantly reminded him of past shortcomings. This "voice" never spoke of anything good or pleasant or funny; the voice delighted only in his pain. It needed to be silenced, he thought, removing the items from his pack. His movements were impulsive, swift, determined.

The alcohol, paint thinner, and blood loss conspired against his senses: His vision blurred, his thoughts subsided, and his sensations went numb. Matt lay down on a rock and fell asleep. Next to him was the empty whiskey bottle and half-empty can of paint thinner; beside these, blood pooled around the razor blade, a shimmering island of steel in a sea of red.

Matt did not know how long he lay there before he awoke. A familiar cold chill had set in over his body. Opening his eyes, he could see the last glimpse of daylight shining through the trees. Again, for reasons only he can know, Matt found the will to live. With slow, trembling hands, he raised himself off the rock. Then he began the mile-long hike back to his car. Often, his vision would blur, and he would fall to his knees while he regained his strength. He was a soul dragging a body, desperately wanting to go on. Matt eventually made it back to his car, and somehow managed to drive himself to the emergency room.

His clothes were filthy and caked in blood as he stumbled into the ER. Upon opening the door, he stammered "suicide attempt." The sight of him alone was all that the receptionist needed; Matt was immediately escorted past triage and into a bed. After three bags of rapid IV fluids, he slowly regained some lucidity. He required numerous stitches on multiple lacerations. When his parents arrived, Matt could not look them in the eyes. He was overwhelmed by feelings of regret, remorse, and guilt.

Matt spent two days on the medicine ward, during which he had to struggle against weakness and fatigue to rise out of bed. A nurse sat in his room on a twenty-four-hour suicide watch. This was the low point in his struggle with bipolar disorder; the memory of it for a time motivated him to continue treatment. After his stay on medicine, Matt was transferred to the psychiatry unit. The psychiatrist there, also a military academy graduate, developed a good rapport with Matt. His no-nonsense, "damn it, take your medicine" approach worked.

Matt stabilized on lithium, at least for a time.

The day before she left the hospital, Lisa finally told me about her suicide attempt with a plastic bag. "I lay on the floor of my dorm room," she said slowly, then she went on to recount the details of her method. She had suffered a sort of mental suffocation for so long, and this act mirrored her mental state. But at the last moment, she changed her mind, and she did not allow her lungs to suffocate as well. "I was so ashamed," she continued. "You are the only person I have ever told."

I paused. "It is good you were able to talk about it."

"Yes. I know."

Lisa was discharged from the hospital the following day. Since the lithium plan had run into a snag, we had done little for her medically in the hospital other than keep her safe. She was to follow up on the second set of kidney tests and hopefully re-start the medication as an outpatient. Despite our lack of intervention, her depression had lifted enough to allow her to safely leave the hospital.

While in the hospital, she wrote:

> My doctor asked me why I think my illness went away without a change of medication in the hospital—how my moods spontaneously stabilized. My answer will certainly not hold up in a medical court of law. I do not think it was the solitude of hospitalization or a special source of willpower. I think it's because it is meant to happen this way. I was meant to have this experience and one day it will be exactly clear why.

Not long after, I received an unexpected email from Lisa, who congratulated me on my recent graduation from medical school and updated me on her progress. Her kidneys were healthy, and she did get back on the lithium, which had since helped stabilize her moods. She was feeling better and was studying to be a psychiatric nurse practitioner.

She desired to help others afflicted, as she is, with mental illness. I replied to her message and asked her permission to tell her story here, changing only her name to protect her identity. She granted permission, writing:

> At first, you want to keep the knowledge of your illness hidden tight inside where no one can see it. It isn't a visible disability, so it is easy to fool most people until things get really bad. But then, when you are well, you want others to understand what you went through, to stop it from being something taboo, something your parents have to lie to their coworkers about and something you should keep secret from your grandparents.

Matt also wanted his story told for similar reasons. He wanted others to understand the suffering and pain associated with his illness, which few people around him could comprehend.

The act of giving a person a diagnostic label can be both stigmatizing and freeing. This is particularly true for mental illness. The diagnostic tag can be abused, as when the physician reduces another person—a complete life in all its richness—to a mere disease or disorder. On the other hand, a diagnosis can be liberating for patients. It can help explain experiences that otherwise remain baffling. We do well to remember that patients are much more than their disease; they are people with talents, hopes, and struggles, who also happen to have bipolar illness.

These two people—one a friend, the other a patient—changed my life and my career. They taught me how to approach the mystery of my patients as individual persons, so as never to reduce them to mere diseases. The best physician will understand his patients both from below, with a sound knowledge of human biology, and from above, with a psychology open to seeing the unique complexity and full story of every patient's life. All the while the physician must remember that these two approaches aim toward, without ever attaining, the invisible horizon where mind and matter, body and soul, meet. Here, the doctor treads on sacred ground. He gazes into a personal abyss whose depths he can never fully plumb.

Matt initiated my interest in becoming a psychiatrist. Lisa convinced me that I had made the right decision. My thoughts echo the sentiments of the protagonist in Walker Percy's novel *The Moviegoer*, who explains his decision to become a doctor: "There is only one thing I can do: Listen to people, see how they stick themselves into the world, hand them along a ways in their dark journey, and be handed along, and for good and selfish reasons."[5]

When Lisa left the hospital, I thought we had failed her, that we had accomplished nothing. I never suspected I would hear from her again. Life sometimes surprises us. While Lisa was my patient, I had tried. Uncertain as I was about the outcome, it was the trying that counted. For us there is only the trying. The rest is not our business.

My wife paged me. "Your mom wants you to call her when you get home," Jennifer said. "She said to call her on her cell." I was standing in a crammed nursing station, filled past capacity with residents, attendings, nurses, and medical students. Now in my second year of residency, I was a licensed physician in the state of California, humming smoothly along my career path. I could barely hear my wife amidst the noise. She also had a buzzing background of noise: Our two sons, ages four and one, were tugging on her pants and asking her questions while she tried to relay the message. "She sounded kind of upset, so don't forget."

"I'll call as soon as I get out of here. I'm trying to wrap up a consult . . . kind of a complicated case. Sorry I'm late home again . . . I'm trying to finish quickly, so I can leave." Jen had heard this before. She understood the life of a resident.

I connected with my mother just as my car merged onto the crowded freeway. It was Friday traffic in the dark. "Why don't you call me again when you get home?" Mom suggested.

But I could hear something in her voice. I would not wait. "Tell me now, Mom."

". . . committed suicide." Was it the static of a bad cell phone connection, or the static of my mind, blocking out what I did not want to hear?

"Who?"

"Matt died by suicide."

My cry was stifled, choked. I do not recall the rest of the hour-long drive home, except that it was dark outside. And inside.

Jennifer opened the door for me when I got home. "Are you okay?" It was plain to her by my expression that I was not.

"No," I shook my head.

She knew before I told her. "Is it Matt?"

"Yes. He killed himself . . ."

She fell into my arms, and I into hers.

Jennifer and I made several phone calls the next day to friends who knew Matt. I called my fellow psychiatry resident and friend, Mark, to ask if he could take my call the following week so that I could fly up for the funeral. Although he did not know my deceased friend, Mark understood better than most. He knew what I was experiencing. It was a feeling familiar to doctors, even young doctors: A physician feels more strongly what he cannot do than what he can.

"He never really accepted the fact of his mental illness," I explained to Mark. "He took lithium for a while but has been off meds for at least a year now. He's been searching for some other medical cause of his symptoms, always doing research on the internet. He would call me every now and again to ask me medical questions. You know, like, 'Do you think it's hypothyroidism?' or 'I think it's just gluten insensitivity: If I don't eat wheat, and exercise a lot, I'll be fine.' He always tried to find some esoteric explanation . . . something other than bipolar."

I continued, "I talked with him on the phone, just two weeks ago. It was the typical questions, and I told him I thought all his symptoms could be accounted for by depression; they were all aspects of his depression, but he wouldn't accept that."

Mark offered some words. He knew what bipolar disorder really entailed; he had seen what it could do to a person. There was some comfort in being understood.

As I spoke to my fellow resident about Matt, I began to feel not just sadness, but anger as well. The anger was not directed toward my deceased friend—no, it was directed toward the disease that claimed his life. I hated mental illness. "At least he's finally free of that demon," was all I could think to say.

We talked on for a few minutes. Then Mark said, "It makes you grateful, to be doing what we do."

"Yeah," I replied. "It's easy to forget what we are really dealing with. You see it when you're on the other side of things." I paused. "It's life and death."

Just a few weeks prior to his death, I had visited my parents in Washington State for Christmas. Matt lived down the street from them. I could not remember the last time I had visited my family without also seeing Matt. But this time was different. We brought a stomach virus with us on the plane, and my parents and siblings all caught it. Not wanting to infect anyone else, I decided to lay low until I felt better. It was then that Matt called me to ask if I wanted to go down to the local pool for a swim while I was in town. I said yes and told him I'd call him in a few days when I was feeling better. I did not call until the day before we left. Matt was not home. I left a message.

I had heard something different in his voice when he initially called to invite me. I did not grasp what it was at the time. Looking back, I think he wanted to go swimming because that is what we used to do together in the summer on the lake where we both grew up. In retrospect, it is now clear: Matt wanted to see me again one final time. He wanted to say goodbye.

We flew out the next day. Matt called me back just as our plane was about to take off. The stewardess asked passengers to turn off all portable electronic devices. "I'll call you when we land," I told Matt. "I'm sorry things didn't work out this time," I said and offered some feeble excuses. "We'll get together next time I'm in town."

Matt said that he understood; he sounded cheerful and forgiving. We spoke on the phone again a week later, but I would never see him again. I did not know it then, but I had missed my last opportunity.

In every one of his prior suicide attempts, there was a core, deep within Matt, that remained untouched by his illness. No matter how overwhelming the effects of his diseased brain, no matter how ruthlessly his illness drove him toward oblivion, in his heart, I am convinced, Matt never really wanted to die. This is clear from the way that he—not just once, but three times—clawed his way heroically back from the brink. I believe this final time was no different. It's just that the means he used were more definitive.

Among all Matt's endearing character traits, one stands out in my mind: his sincerity, his wonder, his delight in the beauty of the world. He never lost the simple gaze of a small boy. Backpacking with a group of high school buddies in the mountains, Matt would sneak up behind someone and pelt him with a snowball. The victim of his ruse would turn to see Matt howling with laughter. For Matt, this prank was hilarious—not just the first time, but also the tenth time. He was so childlike that it was impossible to be irritated as you brushed off the snow. You just shook your head at him and smiled—or better, laughed with him. How had he managed to hold on to the delights that no longer amused the "mature" among us?

Matt relished the natural world. He loved snow, lakes, and rivers. He loved running, fishing, diving, and flying. Through his rigorous military training, through his competitive higher education, through his torturous illness, Matt always remained a wide-eyed boy. And the world was his playground.

The day of his death, my mother spent four hours with Matt's mother, holding her hand. My mom was one of the few in whom Matt confided. He would drop by her office or home every now and again to chat and unburden himself.

I spoke with Matt's mother and brother that night. She told me, "I want you to know, Aaron, that you did everything you could to prevent this. I'm a psychiatric nurse; I knew what he needed. I would beg him, 'Please, Matt, just take a little bit of lithium.' I've seen it work, but he refused." Later she explained, "We had a conversation after his prior suicide attempts. He told us that if he ever harmed himself, it would not be our fault. He told us not to blame ourselves. Matt knew that his family and friends loved him and that he loved us. He wrote a suicide note that said he still loved us, and he loved God, and this did not change that." In our brief conversation, she gave me more consolation than I could possibly have given her. She prayed for me, right there on the phone.

I wished there was more I could have done to help Matt, to help his family. That old feeling still has not left me. As a physician, I feel more strongly what I cannot do than what I can.

I had not always felt powerless to rescue Matt. Several years before, on a mountaineering trip with a group of friends, I did—quite literally—rescue him. One evening, after making camp and pitching our tents, we all agreed to go on a "solo" excursion for the night. We each took our sleeping bags, along with one meal, and ventured off alone, each in a different direction. We settled far enough apart to be unable to see one another or to see the camp. The plan was to sleep alone and return to camp in the morning. I suppose this was a kind of young-man-in-the-wilderness rite of passage.

The plan was thwarted by rain. The weather turned sour just before sundown. Most of us lingered for a few minutes by ourselves, hoping the drizzle would subside. But one by one, we all made our way back to the shelter of the tents while there was still daylight—and before our sleeping gear was soaked through. All of us, that is, except one.

Just as I was drifting off to sleep, our guide asked, "Where's Matt? Did anyone see him come back?"

"Maybe he's in the other tent," someone offered.

I stuck my head out and yelled to our companions, "Is Matt with you guys?"

"No. We figured he was with you," came the reply.

"Damn."

I offered to go look for him. The guide handed me two flashlights as I bundled up. Outside, there was no moon; clouds veiled the stars. The light drizzle had turned into a heavy rain. "I think he went off that way," the guide pointed. "You have ten minutes. If you haven't found him by then, come back. Stay within earshot of the tents. I don't want two people lost out there." I went in the general direction the guide gestured. Before long, I was well beyond earshot of the tents, which was not that far due to the noise of the wind and rain.

"Matt!" I yelled continuously for my friend, with no discernible reply. "Matt!" My voice sounded muffled against the elements.

Finally, I heard, or thought I heard, a faint reply. "Kheriaty . . ." I moved forward, still calling Matt's name. "Kheriaty! I'm down here!" As I shone the flashlight down the hill, Matt's figure came into view. To this day, many years later, I still have a distinct impression of what he looked like at that moment. I can picture him from head to toe. His bare, wiry legs stuck out of the bottom of his blue running shorts. He wore no sweater, fleece, or jacket. He carried no flashlight. He was utterly alone.

This image of Matt has become for me a sort of metaphor for his mental illness. He stood alone—alone in the dark, shivering in the rain. Matt's predicament of bipolar disorder, unlike his predicament on the mountain that night, lasted not just a few hours, but five agonizing years. On the mountain years before, I led him back to camp, back to warmth and light and peaceful sleep. But this time, I could not lead him back—could not really even find him. Perhaps I did not search him out diligently enough. Perhaps I could have done more. Perhaps not.

In any case, I have hope that he is no longer buffeted by the elements—that his air is no longer frigid and dark. The day I learned of Matt's death, words from a favorite poem by Gerard Manley Hopkins kept repeating in my memory:

> *I say that we are wound*
> *With mercy round and round*
> *As if with air . . .*

The poem ends:

> *Stir in my ears, speak there*
> *Of God's love, O live air,*
> *Of patience, penance, prayer:*
> *World-mothering air, air wild,*
> *Wound with thee, in thee isled,*
> *Fold home, fast fold thy child.*[6]

CHAPTER 8

The Receiving End

For he wounds, but he binds up; he smites, but his hands heal.
—Job 5:18[1]

"Aaron, Aaron, Aaron!" My wife saw it coming. I did not. Jennifer was sitting in the passenger seat. I had hastily changed lanes and slowed down, trying to make an exit on an unfamiliar road. The car behind me could not slow down; it hit us with astonishing force. Receiving the blow, our compact car accelerated and began to rotate; we were sliding sideways along the highway. There was no controlling the car now.

Something unexpected happened. My eyes were on my wife through the entire episode: I found myself *above* Jennifer; that is, I was up, and she was down. But I was still in the driver's seat, strapped in, and she was still in the passenger seat. Then just as suddenly, I was no longer above her, and she was no longer below me; we were level, as two people riding in a car ought to be. But we were upside down. Then she was above me, and I was below her. Still not right. Then we were even again, with our heads toward the sky, our feet toward the earth—just right.

But we continued to roll. Without pause, as if in a bad dream, the surreal sequence repeated itself. Finally, we came to rest, our feet closer to the night sky than our heads. We hung there, suspended by our seat belts. Our car had not only rolled; it had rotated, such that we faced the oncoming traffic. I saw white light refracted in a thousand pieces of broken glass; the shattered windshield was a kaleidoscope of shimmering headlights from oncoming traffic. Our car was still running. The radio was still playing. Classical music, I remember.

While we rolled, I could feel a distinct crash each time, as the side, then top, then other side, then wheels slammed the pavement. "Bouncing" is probably a more accurate word than "rolling." Right, up, left, down—my body was slammed in succession. All the while, a single terrifying thought filled my mind: I would live, and she would die. Spare her, Lord. Please. Don't take her. Not now. Not yet.

"Are you okay? Jennifer, are you okay?" I feared that there would be no answer.

"I'm alright."

"Jennifer!"

"I'm okay. I can't move my head. It's stuck."

I reached down, unconsciously, turned off the car and pocketed the key. I have no memory of this, but I found the key in my pocket the next day, so I must have done so. The radio went silent. My hands unclipped the seatbelt and I rolled over, crouching on my hands and knees. There was broken glass everywhere; I brushed shards from my face and eyelashes as I scooted toward Jennifer, who was still hanging upside down.

Her long hair had flown out the broken windshield and was stuck underneath the car—pinned between the car's roof and the pavement. This was why her head could not move, not even an inch: it was jammed in the corner where windshield meets door and window meets ceiling.

The two passengers in the car that hit us ran toward our overturned vehicle. The man shouted to see if we were alive; the woman cried and screamed hysterically.

"We're okay," I said, trying to reassure him and calm her, to no avail. "I need something to cut with. Scissors, a knife, anything."

"I have something in my car," the man said. "I'll be right back."

For some reason, he had a small kitchen knife in his car, which he handed me through the broken window. (To this day, I still have the knife—a little souvenir.) The blade was dull. I began to saw at Jennifer's long, lovely hair.

"I don't care about the hair. We're alive. Do whatever you have to."

I did my best to cut as little hair as possible. Her face close to mine as I sawed, she reassured me, "It's okay. I love you." When her head was free, she unbuckled and maneuvered down onto her hands and knees. I crawled out the rear window, which was also shattered, and made my way to the passenger side where Jennifer was. I was just helping to drag her out of the squished passenger window when the ambulance arrived.

"Don't move her!" the paramedic ordered, pushing me out of the way. They strapped Jennifer on a board and immobilized her neck with a collar. "Was there anyone else in the car?" they asked.

"No, just the two of us," I replied.

The man who pushed me aside had not realized I too was a passenger. "Are you okay?"

"Yeah, I'm fine." I looked down at my hands. They were bleeding. "I'm fine." They made me sign a form that stated I had refused medical attention at the accident scene.

As they were loading Jennifer into the ambulance, I ran back to the car to fetch something I had noticed when I crawled out the back. Our wedding album was lying on the street, behind the car. It must have flown out the back window when the car tumbled and the window shattered. We had been returning from the airport, where we were supposed to have picked up a friend. Jennifer had wanted to show her our wedding pictures, so the album was in the back seat. Our friend's flight had been rerouted to another airport due to inclement weather, so she had fortunately not been in the car with us. The box that held it was broken, but the album itself and the photos inside were intact. I carried it to the ambulance.

"Where are we going?" I asked the driver, as we sped away. "Georgetown?" It was the closest hospital.

"No. George Washington," he replied. GW was the local level one trauma center.

We waited at the hospital for the neck X-rays to come back. Jennifer was still lying immobilized on the hard board with the plastic collar around her neck. The X-ray results were suggestive of a bony abnormality, but the emergency physician thought this could have been a minor congenital anomaly. He paged the radiologist for a second opinion. We would have to wait.

Finally, the radiologist read the film as normal, clearing Jennifer of a spinal injury. They removed her collar. Then, they escorted us into another examining room, where they checked out our eyes with a "slit lamp" to look for corneal abrasions. We picked shards of glass out of our coats for some time, but none of the broken glass had damaged our eyes. We walked out of the hospital that night and caught a cab back to our apartment.

The next day, Valentine's Day, we both stayed home. After our brush with death, we took some time to savor life. That next morning's breakfast tasted splendid. Everything was splendid. We were alive.

But this was only the beginning—the beginning of our year of medical mishaps.

My next mishap earned me a longer stay in the hospital. But first, I want to tell you about what remained of our car.

We went to the junkyard the next day to recover any items left in the car. There was no salvaging the car itself. All the windows, save one, had shattered. To get inside, we had to pry open one of the doors with a crowbar. The roof had folded on impact. Just over the passenger seat there was a sharp edge of triangulated steel pointing down into the car. This was where Jennifer's head would have been, had it not been pinned to the corner by her hair. There, the roof was still intact. When she saw this, my wife cried.

Less than a month later, Jennifer became pregnant with our first child. We like to joke that the accident knocked an egg out of her ovary.

After the car accident, my next mishap occurred that summer while I was visiting my parents. I grew up on a lake in northwest Washington State, and I was glad to return there for a much-needed vacation. Since I was scheduled to fly back to school the following day, I had been trying to squeeze in as much waterskiing as I could. Some friends had come by my parents' house in their boat and invited me to go skiing. I grabbed my wetsuit and jumped in. Already exhausted from one round of skiing and wakeboarding that morning, I foolishly decided to take one last ski.

Slalom waterskiing is a high-speed sport. Cutting across the wake, the skier reaches speeds twice that of the boat. When you hit the water at sixty miles per hour, there is not much cushion. I do not remember the fall that day. My body bent backwards and the back of the ski, without coming off my feet, popped up and struck the right side of my head. My friends later told me that after the fall I had been flopping about in the water; this was likely a seizure due to the head trauma.

I only remember finding myself curled up on the boat seat, looking down at a pool of blood. My head throbbed . . . *blood on my hands . . . hands on my head . . . in a boat . . . what boat? Where?* Confused, tired. *Ouch. My head.* Blood was everywhere. Voices in the background murmured . . . someone was calling 911. The paramedics met us on a nearby dock and dragged my floppy body out of the boat. They cut my wetsuit off my body (*zipper in the back . . . just roll me over . . . don't cut expensive wetsuit*, I remember thinking). Riding in an ambulance . . . lying in the ER . . . my wife and parents peering over me . . . now inside a white tube—a CT scanner . . . someone was yelling at me to hold still, but my head throbbed, and I felt naked and cold, and I could not hold still. *Hold still. Still.*

I woke up that night in a hospital bed.

"Your ear looked like it had gone through a meat grinder," Jennifer later told me. "I didn't think they would be able to salvage it. I kept thinking I was going to have a husband with one ear." I will be ever grateful to the surgeon (coincidentally, already a friend of the family) who put my ear back on my head, sewing the jigsaw puzzle pieces of overlying skin back together with needle and thread. He did what my wife thought could never be done. Today, the scar is barely visible.

I learned some things while on the receiving end of medical and surgical care. A few days in the hospital convinced me that it is not the doctors, but the nurses, who make the time in a hospital manageable or miserable. I realized that hospital food tastes even worse than it looks, that the hospital beds are far more uncomfortable than they appear, and that television is no substitute for human company when you are sick. I saw the lonely, hungry, uncomfortable reality of modern medical care from an entirely different angle. Later, I tried to recall these things as I hurried in and out of patients' rooms, trying to finish the many "important" tasks that need to be completed before the end of the workday, with no time to spare, no time to give the patient the little things they really wanted.

Physicians often have no idea how much a few brief words of encouragement mean to a suffering patient. Although memories tend to fade, I do not want to forget what it is like to be that patient.

I had been washing dishes in the kitchen when the news came.

"I think I'll do another pregnancy test," Jennifer had said.

"You did one last month. Those are not cheap. We should take out stock in pregnancy tests," I teased her.

"I really think I might be." A moment later, "Aaron . . . oh my gosh . . . there's a pink line." I immediately broke out in a sweat. Here we go . . . married with a kid while in med school. This would be a challenge. We were nervous. We were overjoyed.

The pregnancy itself was not the mishap; it was the complications of pregnancy and the emergency delivery. After weeks on and off bed rest for a condition called preeclampsia (elevated blood pressure during pregnancy with risks of seizure during delivery), Jennifer's water broke. Unexpectedly, at three in the morning, and three weeks before her due date, her body began to push the baby out.

Jennifer had wanted to take the "all natural" approach to childbirth: no drugs, no epidural, no episiotomy unless she had no other choice. She suffered through the intense contractions completely painkiller-free for many hours. Despite her determination, she made little progress with labor. Blood labs showed a drop in platelets, which put her at high risk for bleeding during delivery. Her preeclamptic condition had progressed to a rare, more serious condition known as HELLP syndrome—severe preeclampsia with associated rupture of red blood cells, low platelets, and liver damage. The only remedy was delivery. But natural childbirth was nowhere in sight; she was not yet halfway dilated. Every minute counted.

"We have to do a C-section," the obstetrician informed us. We had complete confidence in Dr. Bruchalski, one of the finest doctors I have known.[2] "I don't think she'll be able to deliver in time, and if her platelets continue to drop, she may bleed excessively. We need to get the baby out," he explained.

The anesthesiologist came in to put in the epidural. Before long, Jen's agonized contractions were reduced to a mere elevated line on the monitor. "Am I having one?" she would ask, unable to feel the cramped squeeze of uterine muscle. Anesthesia, what a fine invention.

They wheeled my wife into the operating room. Jennifer fearlessly watched the entire procedure via a mirror above her head as she lay on the operating table. Still in my second year, without much experience with surgeons, I watched in wonder at the rapidity and confidence with which Dr. Bruchalski wielded the scalpel. In minutes, his hands were inside, searching for our baby. We watched in anticipation. "It's a boy," he announced, pulling out a gray, goopy little guy. "What's his name?"

"His name is John," I replied.

The two doctors in the room—both named John—gave an approving cheer.

Jennifer saw our son for a few moments, as I held him near her face, before the anesthesiologist turned up the juice and she drifted off to sleep. While the doctors closed her up, a nurse escorted me to another room, where John—less than five pounds, but healthy—was placed under a heating lamp. It would be many hours before Jennifer awoke. I sat alone with my firstborn child staring at his tiny body.

Only later did I realize how serious Jennifer's condition had been. Only later did I fully understand that she could very well have died.

During morning rounds on my obstetrics rotation one year later, I was presenting my first patient, a thirty-year-old woman having her first child. Like Jennifer, the late stages of her pregnancy were complicated by preeclampsia; like Jennifer, she had developed HELLP syndrome in the hospital while in labor; and like Jennifer, she had gone into labor four weeks early, trying unsuccessfully to deliver her firstborn the natural way.

"Why did they do a C-section?" the attending asked. "Is HELLP syndrome an indication for cesarean?"

"Not necessarily," I answered, correctly. "But her platelets were dropping, and this put her at risk of bleeding."

"But bleeding risk may be a contraindication to surgery," the attending countered.

Undeterred, I went on, "Yes, but she likely had many hours to go in labor, and her platelets would continue to drop until she delivered. This would put her at higher risk of vaginal or uterine bleeding after delivery."

"Right . . . good," the attending said. I continued to field his pimp questions until he had exhausted the subject of HELLP syndrome. This was my hour to shine: the one obstetric condition that I knew a lot about. The residents were impressed. I didn't tell them how I knew so much.

I vividly remember this delivery, the first that I assisted on. Before making my way to the scrub station, I had found a few moments to explain to the patient what Jennifer had gone through. Sensing her fear—for her baby as well as for herself—I explained that my wife had endured a similar first delivery. I told her that John was born three weeks early and was now a bouncing one-year-old, and that Jennifer had recovered fully in due time. Her husband seemed equally relieved to hear my story. My experience in obstetrics was extremely limited, but I did know something about their situation.

The patient recovered well. Her baby did not fare quite as well as John, spending several weeks in the neonatal intensive care unit, but eventually the boy went home healthy. The mom spent every day at the hospital with her baby. After I had finished obstetrics and had moved on to another rotation, I would see her there from time to time. She would update me on her baby's progress and thank me for my help while she was in the hospital. I had done little for her medical care, except for waking her up at six in the morning during my pre-rounds. The doctors had saved her and her baby's life. I had merely sympathized and understood, but for her, that was meaningful.

Six months after John was born, I received an unexpected phone call. I was enjoying a weekend away from the demands of school and family life on a retreat. My hours of quiet contemplation were interrupted by the sound of my wife's voice on the other end. "John broke his leg. We're at the hospital. I was carrying him down the back stairs, with the laundry in my other hand, and . . . I fell," Jennifer confessed.

"Are you hurt?"

"Just bruised, nothing broken. Aaron, I'm so sorry . . ." She burst into tears.

"It's not your fault. It was an accident." Jennifer had retold her story many times to various hospital personnel. Doctors and nurses kept asking her to repeat it, trying to ascertain whether the incident was truly an accident. They compared notes and found no inconsistencies.

A nurse warned her that social services might come by the house to ask the same questions, just to make sure. The ugly truth is that pediatricians see too many broken limbs of children that are not accidental.

"Which hospital are you at?"

"Georgetown."

"I'll leave now. It will take me a few hours to get back to DC."

The X-ray showed a clean break of the femur. It was not a spiral fracture, which is considered child abuse until proven otherwise, because this type of break almost invariably occurs by grabbing and twisting with two hands. By the time I arrived, both John's legs were in a sling, bent at the knees. We spent the night on the pediatric ward. The team of medical students, residents, and the physician making rounds woke us early the next morning. They stayed in the room less than a minute and never once addressed me.

John was immobilized in the sling for the next four weeks, which seemed like a long time for a little guy who was so fond of crawling. Babies' bodies, although they appear fragile, are remarkably resilient. They heal more rapidly than the rest of us. Jen's psychological scars, the guilt of falling while carrying him, took longer to heal.

One evening in the emergency room two years later: "Eight-month-old boy, rule out skull fracture," the resident said. "You want to go see this one?"

"Sure," I replied, taking the chart from her. I glanced through the triage nurse's note. It looked familiar.

I walked into the examining room, where a mother was holding her baby boy. "Could you tell me what happened?" I asked her, already knowing the answer. This was probably the third or fourth time the mother had explained it since they arrived at the hospital.

"I was carrying him down the stairs," she began, but hesitated. She glanced at me furtively. There was a look of shame and anguish on her face. "I . . . I fell down, and I think he hit his head." My gut told me that she, like my wife two years prior, was telling the truth.

I put my hand on her shoulder. "My wife fell down the stairs with our son when he was six months old. He broke his leg. I know you've gone over this story many times already. Don't worry."

She let out a sigh of relief and smiled at me. "Thank you."

I warned her about the possibility of questioning from child protective services, that this was routine and that she was not necessarily being accused of anything. She thanked me again.

"Now, let me have a look," I said. She handed me the boy. I examined the back of his skull as I held him. There was some swelling.

"Do you think we need an X-ray?" the attending asked me, after I presented the case.

"It wouldn't hurt. There may be a minor skull fracture."

"How likely is this?"

"Not very," I surmised.

"What could we do if there was one?"

"Nothing."

"Right. Let's get the films anyway. You could go either way on this, but it's nice to know for sure."

The X-ray did show a minor fracture of the skull. I returned to the examining room and explained this to the mother. She began crying again. "This will heal on its own," I said. "There's nothing we need to do for it, since the bone is not displaced." I tried to reassure her. "These babies appear fragile, but they are really very resilient. They bounce back so quickly." She thanked me one last time, and I walked out of the room.

I have told the story of John's broken leg to many friends and family members, all of whom seem to have some similar story to tell: "You know, I fell off my changing table when I was a year old," or "My mom dropped my little sister, and she turned out all right." My favorite anecdote was from a guy whose brother was tossing his little baby in the air and catching him. Not paying attention, the father tossed the boy too close to a whirring ceiling fan; the poor lad was thumped square in the forehead with the fan blade. He bled a bit from the cut but there was no permanent damage. After hearing that story, Jennifer did not feel so bad about her accidental fall.

After John broke his leg, my father came to visit. His intention was to help out while I was busy with finals. Instead, my father also ended up in Georgetown Hospital.

The day after arriving, he began to have abdominal cramps, fever, and diarrhea. When I got home from school, he was lying on the couch after spending much of the day in the bathroom. Lounging around was not my dad's usual mode of operation, so I knew immediately that something was amiss. He minimized the discomfort, insisting that he probably ate something bad and would likely feel better soon. But a few hours later, he suggested, ever so furtively, that maybe he might benefit from a trip to the ER. I knew then without a doubt that something was really wrong. My father, like many stoic men, does not voluntarily go to the doctor unless absolutely necessary, much less the emergency room.

I took a brief "history" of his symptoms and palpated his abdomen, pretending like I knew what I was doing. "Any tenderness when I press down?" I asked. I even listened to his bowel sounds with a stethoscope, although I did not know the significance of what I was hearing. "I think it might be diverticulitis," I told him.

"What does that mean?"

"As people get older, most develop little outpouchings in the colon called diverticula. They're usually not a problem, unless they get infected. With diverticulitis, you need antibiotics. The docs will probably want to scope you, to have a look at the colon."

"Great," he groaned sarcastically, frowning at the prospect of a fiber-optic scope in the rectum.

The emergency room physician agreed with my diagnostic guess. (I was still a second-year student without clinical experience, so calling this a "guess" is accurate.) He indeed ordered a colonoscopy, which showed non-specific inflammation of the colon, but not diverticulitis. My father was admitted to the hospital to receive antibiotics and hydration through an IV.

I came to visit him after class the next day. He told me about the troop of med students, residents, and the attending physician who came by early that morning to examine him and discuss his diagnosis, the exact nature of which was still a mystery. Although he was not a man who liked lying in a hospital gown before a large group of people talking about his bowel habits, he was a good sport about it.

"I knew that this would be you next year," he told me. His kindness to the third-year student paid off a few days later. "This morning, the attending told me I could go home today," he told the student. "But all afternoon, he was nowhere to be found. No one seems to know anything about my discharge." The med student finally took pity on him and ran around getting the paperwork in order and obtaining the appropriate signatures so that he could go home.

They never figured out the exact cause of my father's colitis. The inflammation and symptoms resolved with antibiotics. Although he was in the hospital for five days, I was relieved that this family member's stay at Georgetown was mostly uneventful. On the other hand, I wondered if our ill fortune might be rubbing off on visitors. Were our medical mishaps becoming contagious?

Years later, a decade into my career as an attending physician, I suffered from a chronic pain condition that lasted nearly five years. A lumbar disk rupture led to incapacitating pain, followed by two spine surgeries that failed to resolve the pain. I could only sit or stand for an hour or so before I needed to lay down to relieve the pain. I wouldn't wish this kind of injury on my worst enemy. But I will say that it's not a bad thing for physicians, from time to time, to also be on the receiving end of medical care. You see things differently when you're lying on the examination table.

During that time, I saw physical rehab docs, pain docs, four spine surgeons—all of them excellent, though none of them successful with my case. Even before we embarked on the project of trying to find a solution, I needed the physician to acknowledge the implications of the disease. One of the most consoling encounters with a doctor I had during this time took only a moment. It was so subtle that most people wouldn't have noticed. I was seeing a top-flight spine surgeon at UC Irvine. After looking at the MRI of my original injury and severe nerve compression, he paused for a few seconds before launching into his assessment and recommendations. He took a moment just to acknowledge the severity of my pain, to sit with it, without immediately trying to jump in and fix it.

As it turned out, he couldn't fix the problem, but that was okay. In that moment of acknowledgment and recognition, his humanity shined through. A physician's knowledge and technical competence are necessary but never sufficient. The doctor cares for the patient primarily by *caring* for the patient. It is disarmingly simple, yet often challenging, especially when we are overworked, or stressed, or fatigued: to forget about yourself and give yourself generously to the patient in front of you.

One night on call during my final year of medical school, although I was not a patient this time, I slept on the psychiatry ward with the patients. This was the first year they had an acting internship in psychiatry, and they had neglected to secure a call room for us. The first few times on call, I brought a camping pad and slept on the floor in the psychiatric day hospital wing, where there were no patients at night. This was a bit absurd, but what is an exhausted medical student to do?

That night, I asked the charge nurse where I could find fresh sheets and a blanket. He asked me where I had been sleeping.

"Across the hall in the group therapy room."

Another nurse stopped me. "I wouldn't sleep over there, especially not on the floor. There are cockroaches."

Cockroaches? In a hospital? "I have to sleep on the floor. The couch over there is way too short for me," I responded.

"Why don't you just sleep here on the psych ward in one of the empty patient rooms?" the night nurse suggested. "I'll tell the nurse in the morning not to bother you."

"Is that allowed?" I asked. The prospect of sleeping in a room next to psychotic patients did not interest me, but I was getting tired. After several nights sleeping on the floor, a hospital bed sounded pretty appealing.

"It's fine with me," the nurse replied. "Probably against policy, but what the hell." It was also against policy for the hospital not to have a call room for me. Either way, I was breaking the rules.

So I did: I slept in the locked psych unit. The night nurse must have forgotten to tell the next shift's nurse that I was there, because he woke me up the next morning for a suicide assessment check. I explained that I was the acting intern, not a patient. Probably assuming that I was just another delusional patient, the nurse apologized anyway, turned off the light, and closed the door.

It was the best night of sleep I had on call.

In my first few years of medical training, I learned some valuable things about being a physician. More importantly, in those years I also learned a few things about being a patient, or a patient's loved one—about what it means to be in the sick role. These were, in some respects, harder lessons: the firsthand experience of illness and its attendant helplessness, the frustrations of navigating our byzantine healthcare system, the anxiety of watching a loved one suffer. I hope they have made me a more empathetic healer. Without these experiences, I probably would have drifted away from my patients, assuming the character of the distant doctor who has forgotten what it means to first be a human being.

To understand medicine at the deepest level, we must start not with looking at what doctors do, and not with looking at medical technologies or techniques; we must start with patients—with the existential experience of illness. Disease and disability are universal features of human life, potentially striking any person—young or old, rich or poor, famous or obscure—at any time, often through no fault of their own. From the beginning, society has always needed those who are designated to heal. And society confers benefits and privileges on them not accorded to others, like monopolies on prescribing privileges or the license to perform surgery without being thrown in jail. I was permitted to do things in medical school, like practice unperfected procedural skills on patients or carve up a dead body, which would be considered felonies in any other context. The state granted these privileges not for my sake but for the sake of my current and future patients.

Imagine, God forbid, that you wake up tomorrow morning with acute lower abdominal pain, which grows progressively worse despite your efforts to remedy it. Like most people, your first inclination will probably not be to go to the ER or urgent care clinic. You may first try some over-the-counter remedy, perhaps do an internet search based upon your symptoms.

But as the symptoms grow worse, you realize you won't be going to work or school today; perhaps the best you can do now is lay in bed and pray for relief. So your plans are disrupted, and your functionality is impaired. And you are likely growing anxious and fearful: What if this is serious or life-threatening? You realize after some online reading that even if you could diagnose the problem—is this an inflamed gallbladder or appendicitis?—you do not have the means or ability to treat it yourself. So against your inclination, and contrary to your preferences, you call a friend or an ambulance and have them bring you to the emergency room.

When you arrive, you wait in triage longer than you should. Then you are wheeled back on a gurney to a room where a nurse greets you and tells you to remove all your clothes and put on a gown that doesn't entirely close in the back. Perhaps, if they believe you are not malingering, they will administer some narcotics to take the edge off your progressively worsening pain. A doctor arrives—a person you have never met—and introduces herself with the greeting, "How can I help you?" In these circumstances, you had no opportunity to vet the doctor who happened to be on shift that day. You must trust the medical credentialing system sufficiently to believe that perhaps she possesses the requisite knowledge and skills to help you. At that moment, you the patient enter into a relationship of a particular kind with this physician. I'll return to that relationship in a moment.

This doctor, with your implied or explicit consent, then asks you sensitive and personal questions about your bowel habits and your sexual history. She pokes and prods you with a physical exam that focuses especially on the part of the body that hurts the most. Then she sends you down the hall to get stuck with a needle for a blood draw, then to the other end of the hall to be exposed to radiation in the CT scanner, during which she disappears and does not return for a long time, while you wait in anxious anticipation for her diagnostic findings.

Now, why would any sane person subject himself to this kind of ordeal? You do so not because you *want* to, but in a sense, because you *have* to. Acute illness has rendered you vulnerable. You're in pain, nonfunctional, and scared; your life and your plans have been disrupted, and you likely cannot recover without help from a doctor. So, when she offers to help, you accept, opening yourself up to all the inconveniences and indignities this entails. And this situation creates a particular kind of relationship between you as the patient and your new physician who professes to heal.

The first thing to notice about this asymmetrical relationship is the imbalance of power. The doctor and patient are equal in dignity, equal in rights, equal before the law, and so forth. But there is an inequality of power. If things go sideways, you stand to lose much more than the doctor. The necessary ingredient to make this doctor-patient work is therefore trust. I used to tell students that virtually all principles of medical ethics can be distilled in this one precept: to remain worthy of trust, to remain faithful to the trust the patient has placed in you, to act so as to inspire the patient's trust and to avoid doing anything that might undermine this trust.

In legal terms, we call this a fiduciary relationship—from the Latin word *fides*, from which we get the word "faith" or trust. When they hear the word "infidelity," most people think first of cheating in a relationship or adultery in a marriage. Such actions are harmful not primarily because they breach a contract, but because they undermine the trust upon which this kind of relationship is founded: Marriage is the prototypical fiduciary relationship, grounded in trust and requiring fidelity above all else.

My mentor at Georgetown, Dr. Pellegrino, enumerated some of the most essential virtues for physicians as follows:

> (1) Fidelity to trust, which is ineradicable in healing relationships; (2) some suppression of self-interest, since the person served is in a vulnerable state and dependent on the power of the professional; (3) intellectual honesty, since professional practice beyond one's expertise is injurious; (4) compassion, since understanding and feeling something of the unique predicament of the person's need is essential to healing; (5) courage to pursue the good in the face of today's commercialization, depersonalization, and industrialization of professional life; and (6) prudence in every act so that the measures chosen are best suited to the technical and moral good of the person served.[3]

The patient needs to know that the doctor will place all her knowledge and skills always and only at the service of health and healing—that she will do her best to treat the illness, or at list mitigate symptoms where cure is impossible, and that she will minimize harms. As the original Hippocratic Oath professes, "I will follow that system or regimen which according to my ability and judgment I consider for the benefit of my patient and abstain from whatever is deleterious and mischievous." The patient needs to know that the doctor will avoid acting according to external interests or inducements, whether financial, personal, or otherwise—that she will treat the patient the same as she would any other person in the same medical circumstances, regardless of creed, race, status, or any other factor external to the illness. Without this confidence in the doctor's abilities and intentions, trust is undermined, and healing becomes impossible.

Naturally, like every relationship, this one is a two-way street. Doctors bear the bulk of responsibilities due to the imbalance of power, but patients are not without their own responsibilities. For example, patients have the duty to tell the truth and to treat the physician with a minimum level of decency and respect. I recall a consult we received when I chaired the ethics committee at UCI from a plastic surgeon working on our burn unit. She asked if she was ethically required to continue seeing a patient who was mistreating her. When she would enter the patient's room, he would bite off a piece of his gangrenous finger and spit it at her. My answer was no, you do not have a moral responsibly to continue treating this patient. His vulnerability does not grant him license to abuse you. Even very sick patients are capable of civility.

This doctor-patient relationship forms the core of medicine. The nature of this relationship will never change—even with advances in science and technology—because the nature of illness and its effects on human life will not change. But this fiduciary model of medicine is now under assault, with internal and external forces undermining it and pushing new models for medicine—models that will, in the end, only harm vulnerable patients.

Some want to recharacterize the doctor-patient relationship along contractual lines, where the terms of this relationship are negotiated by two fully autonomous agents, with the doctor as a kind of technical assistant available to fulfill the patient's requests. While this may sound attractive at first glance, congenial to our rugged American individualism and our notions of equality, the model sets up patients for failure. Because someone who is rendered vulnerable by illness does not have equal power to simply walk away from the negotiating table if he does not like the terms of the contract. Lying on the hospital gurney, doubled over in the fetal position in pain, is not a good negotiating position: Your viable options are limited. This is why, on this model, the physician's will or preferences will typically prevail. While it appears to start with an assumption of equality, it ends in de facto medical paternalism.

Others are pushing for a consumer- or market-based model for medicine. One can hear this in subtle but significant shifts in language: Physicians become "providers" and patients become "clients" or "consumers" of healthcare services. But like the negotiated contractual model, the consumer model of medicine mischaracterizes the nature of the doctor-patient relationship. In a market, the consumer has most of the power: I can buy what you are selling, or I can go to another seller if I don't like the items in your store, or I can choose to not buy anything at all. Hence the conventional adage in sales that the customer is always right.

But of course, if you are afflicted with acute appendicitis and need to go under the surgeon's knife to save your life, you are not in the power position of a customer buying optional goods and services on the free market. It's hard to shop around for a better deal when you are doubled over in pain. The existential state of illness, and the stakes of bad treatment or no treatment, do not permit this kind of consumer freedom. This is not to deny that medical institutions operate with relevant business principles, much less to deny that market forces influence medicine profoundly, but simply to clarify that the market model is not at the heart of the enterprise. Medical care cannot be reduced to just another market commodity.

The key features of the doctor-patient relationship form the root from which the practice of good medicine must arise: the vulnerability of the sick patient, the inequality of power, the fiduciary character of the relationship, the fact that the knowledge and skills of the physician are not wholly proprietary but are granted for the sake of the sick patient, and the fact that the physician is the locus of responsibility for the medical team. The doctor is the final common pathway through which help or harm comes to the patient.

As such, the physician is also a member of a moral community of other physicians, responsible for holding one another accountable to the high ethical and technical standards of the profession. As a doctor, I am primarily responsible for my own patients; but to a lesser extent, I am also responsible for my colleagues' patients. This is the basis of the requirement in the AMA's Principles of Medical Ethics that, as a member of this professional moral community, I report fellow physicians who are deficient in character or competence—something that is not easy in practice but that is quite reasonably expected by the public, who must trust not just individual physicians but also the profession as a whole.

This is also the basis for the traditional prohibitions, maintained by professional medical societies like the AMA, against physicians using their knowledge and skills for anything other than health and healing. For example, the AMA does not take a position on the ethics of capital punishment itself, but it does say to members that, *as physicians*, they are prohibited from participating in lethal injections or other forms of state-sanctioned killing. Likewise, doctors should not participate in the torture of political prisoners. Traditional prohibitions against assisted suicide and euthanasia follow the same logic: Firefighters should not burn down buildings, even if their expertise could facilitate this, as they do in the dystopian novel *Fahrenheit 451*. The physician who doubles as a part-time executioner, or who moonlights at Guantanamo, undermines the public's trust in medicine as an enterprise exclusively devoted to healing the sick.

The primary goods intrinsic to the practice of medicine, for which the moral community of physicians is responsible, are clear: the healing of individual patients, curing when possible, containing and mitigating illness when cure is impossible, and caring in ways aimed always and only at the promotion of health. These primary goods remain in tension with secondary goods—money, power, prestige, honor, ranking, competitive advantage—which are central to the *institutions* of medicine, such as hospitals, clinics, and medical centers. These dialectical tensions between physicians and institutions are inevitable: A hospital that does not attend to money will squander its financial solvency and no longer be available to support the healing work of doctors. But when the institutional goals of money, prestige, and power threaten to undermine the primary goods of patient care, health, and healing, then physicians have a responsibility to collectively push back for the good of their patients.

Medical professionals and the institutions that support them will always remain in tension. But today, the overwhelming control and power of these institutions now seriously threaten the practice of good medicine. There are strong forces at work today—financial, institutional, and philosophical—attempting to transform medicine from the Hippocratic model of fiduciary care to a technocratic, contractual, market-based, or consumer-driven model that fails to serve the deepest needs of those made vulnerable by disease. Restoring the doctor-patient relationship to the center of the medical enterprise is our best and only cure—a proposition that will require serious reforms of our medical institutions. I will say more about this in the closing chapters.

As I was gaining unasked-for experience being a patient, I was also gradually growing in my comfort with being a doctor. There were still tough days, to be sure, characterized by the typical confusion and bewilderment of a rookie. But there were also a growing number of good days on the wards, when the scrubs and white coat were starting to wear well. There were even a few days of downright bliss.

Leo Tolstoy's novel *Anna Karenina* contains a celebrated passage on the sublime potential of human work. This agrarian scene of a farmer reaping is a beautifully romantic description of a worker lost in his work, totally yet effortlessly absorbed in the task at hand:

> The longer Levin went on mowing, the oftener he experienced those moments of oblivion when his arms no longer seemed to swing the scythe, but the scythe itself his whole body, so conscious and full of life; and as if by magic, regularly and definitely without a thought being given to it, the work accomplished itself of its own accord. These were blessed moments.[4]

There were some days—and even nights on call—on the hospital wards when I experienced these moments of oblivion, wielding not a scythe but a stethoscope. During those times, when I too felt so conscious and full of life, the work of a medical student, as if by magic, seemed to accomplish itself. Those were days when time passed without my noticing. Suddenly, I would discover that it was time to go home. *Optima dies, prima fugit*, said Virgil: "The best of days are the first to flee." However, like the farmer in Tolstoy's novel, these "blessed moments" of effortless work were the exception rather than the rule.

There were other days—and especially other nights—filled with doubt and drudgery, frustration and fatigue, when, far from accomplishing itself of its own accord, all of the work down to the smallest task seemed to be accomplished only with great effort. Even more common than both these extremes were the typical quotidian days, when the work was toilsome but not troublesome and when the ordinary routine was seasoned with small rewards—the everyday toil sprinkled with tiny triumphs.

The beauty of those few blissful days, when work was effortless and I was in a state of flow, covered the ugliness of the dreadful days, and lent added color to the ordinary days. When I began medical school, I was not entirely convinced that I had made the right decision.

Relieved from the burdens of frequent self-consciousness and occasional self-doubt, those few idyllic days of medical work convinced me of what I had hoped was true when I began: Although there had been no stethoscope in my crib, I was indeed meant to be a physician.

One day during transplant surgery rounds with Dr. Katz, she had been grilling us with pimp questions, none of which anyone answered correctly. In a pleasant mood that day, she decided to poke fun at us rather than berate us. "Where ignorance is bliss . . ." she said, waiting for us to finish the line. "Where ignorance is bliss . . ." she repeated. We stood by dumbly. "What's the rest of the line?" she asked, annoyed at our ignorance not only of surgery but also of poetry. "Wasn't anyone here an English major in college?"

"I was," said the resident meekly. "But I don't remember the poem."

Rule number four: If you do not know the answer to a pimp question, look it up that night. So I did a search for "where ignorance is bliss," and found the entire poem. The next day during rounds, I triumphantly announced, "'Where ignorance is bliss, 'tis folly to be wise.' Thomas Gray, eighteenth century American poet."

Dr. Katz smiled at me for the first time. My confidence bolstered by this small victory, I continued, "I thought of a better line of poetry to describe this rotation. It comes from a poem by Robert Frost, 'Stopping by Woods on a Snowy Evening.'"

"Oh yeah, what is it?" Dr. Katz asked.

"'And miles to go before I sleep, and miles to go before I sleep,'" I said, thinking myself quite witty.

"Just remember," she said, now more seriously, "no matter how long you stay here at the hospital, you eventually get to go home. But the patients do not get to go home. They are still stuck here."

"Yeah, it's no fun being sick," the resident mused pensively.

I felt a twinge of shame. At times, blinded by my own self-pity, I forgot the most important thing. Yes, I was tired. Yes, I was overworked. But by comparison, this was nothing. Feeling sorry for myself, I had lost sight of the patients—the ones who were really suffering. How easy it is to forget the most obvious truths: It is no fun being sick.

CHAPTER 9

Quiet Desperation

I have stood here before inside the pouring rain
With the world turning circles running 'round my brain
I guess I'm always hoping that you'll end this reign
But it's my destiny to be the king of pain
　　　　　　　—The Police, "King of Pain"[1]

"The growing good of the world is partly dependent on unhistoric acts," George Eliot wrote in *Middlemarch*. Eliot could have been describing the work of our best physicians rather than her novel's heroine: "And that things are not so ill with you and me as they might have been, is half owing to the number who lived faithfully a hidden life, and rest in unvisited tombs."[2] Whatever prestige still remains attached to this profession, a doctor's life remains mostly a hidden life. And we will, all of us, eventually rest in unvisited tombs.

I had almost no idea what I was getting into when I entered medical school. There were surprises in store, both gruesome and gratifying. During the clinical years, I learned that the physician does what needs to be done for the patient. He may not like it. But he does not recoil or refuse. Much of it was not quite the deft and dignified labor of healing that I had pictured. But eventually, I came to see that a physician's best work is typically inglorious; it usually passes unnoticed. Litigants are all too ready to pounce should the doctor make a mistake (and sometimes even when he does not make a mistake). Few notice when he does his work well. His successes are unheralded, his failures magnified. I grew to accept this fact and try to live faithfully a hidden life.

Even more than doctors, patients live a hidden life, their anguish often invisible even to those closest to them. Henry David Thoreau claimed that most men lead lives of quiet desperation. I cannot judge whether Thoreau spoke truly in his assessment of most men; but I can think of no better description for the state of so many who lie in a hospital bed. Quiet desperation.

As a medical student, and as a physician, I witnessed intense suffering daily. I could not wholly comprehend it. The weight of pain borne by sick patients was, in the last analysis, unfathomable.

Compassion. This is what we were continually urged to cultivate as physicians. Beginning in year one of medical school, we heard frequent admonitions on the need for empathy, understanding, warmth, and compassion. These words probably conjure a picture of a kind-hearted doctor, one who has a good "bedside manner," someone who tries to care for "the whole person." We expect the compassionate physician to feel pangs of emotion—perhaps sadness or grief—for his suffering patients. The compassionate physician will speak to patients in reassuring tones, will perhaps hold their hand, will not abandon them when death is near.

This is all well and good, but it is not sufficient. The Latin root of "com-passion" literally means to "suffer with." We should pause here, for this seems to be asking too much. How is it possible for even the best physician to suffer with his patients? Will he not be overwhelmed by the burden of this task? Is it not better to remain detached, so that he can continue to care for the sick without being engulfed in their pain? I am still searching for answers to these questions after twenty years in practice.

Pain is an unrelenting weight. I have seen it crush strong men and strong women. There were times when it crushed me. I have seen others, who appear frail and fragile, bear its weight serenely, even heroically.

When confronted with heavy suffering, the physician has a choice. He can ignore it, even while acknowledging its presence. It's all around him in the patients he treats, but should he consider their suffering too long or too deeply, it may begin to crush him as well. Perhaps it's better not to think about it. After all, he must continue to work, to do what he can to alleviate the patient's pain. Surely his job is to mitigate suffering, not to *suffer with* the patient. This seems like the reasonable approach to the problem.

Alternatively, he can acknowledge suffering and grant suffering its full weight. He can perhaps even search for some meaning in suffering. To many, this will sound absurd. But is it? To ignore suffering is to court callousness. To declare that it is meaningless and absurd is to flirt with nihilism and despair. The so-called "problem of evil" has vexed philosophers and theologians for millennia, and doubtless vexed ordinary people since the beginning of time. Perhaps "mystery" is a better word than "problem" for the experience of human suffering.

Like everyone else, I certainly have no easy solution to the problem and have found no pat answers to the mystery. Perhaps here, as we explore the meaning of medicine and its attendant dangers, it is enough for me to acknowledge and reflect upon some of the suffering patients I first encountered in medical school.

Mr. Bernanos's head was exploding. We did not know why. He lay in a bed on the neurology service, suffering constant headaches, the worst I had ever encountered. We commonly asked patients to rate their pain on a scale of zero to ten—ten being the worst pain imaginable, zero being no pain. Many patients clearly exaggerated their symptoms in search of opiates, but I could see Mr. Bernanos did not. His headache was consistently an eight or nine, and after heavy pain medications, a five or six. It never went away. Day after day, hour after hour, his head exploded. He could not sleep.

Mr. Bernanos had a history of cancer in his neck. Along with the cancer, his vocal cords had been surgically removed. Lacking these, he could not speak, so he communicated with pencil and paper. Desperately quiet, quietly desperate. We would ask questions, and he would jot down brief answers. "No sleep," rubbing his eyes. "Head hurts, both sides," pointing to his temples. "Eight or nine. More Fentanyl?"

His Fentanyl patch and IV narcotics provided a bit of relief, but even these "big guns" were insufficient. Most chronic pain is manageable with the right regimen, but Mr. Bernanos's headaches remained intractable despite our efforts. We did not know the cause of his headaches, even after numerous tests and imaging studies. Perhaps the cancer had returned and was affecting blood flow to the brain, we wondered? He certainly had the wasting look of a man with cancer.

"He's a priest, you know," the nurse told me one day. "Former Air Force chaplain."

I did not know that. Father Bernanos was not a patient of mine, but I walked by his room every day on the way to the office across the hall. His door was always open, and he would sometimes gesture to me to come in, asking for something with pencil, paper, and hand gesticulations—more pain meds, a pill to help him sleep. I wanted to give him something, but these things he requested were not much help.

A priest, hanging on the Cross with his Lord. His hands, which had so often held the consecrated flesh and blood of Christ, now held his own throbbing head—his own painful flesh and pulsating blood. His voice, which had absolved so many sinners in the confessional, was now mute—never again to speak those sweet words of absolution. Yet he remained what he was, even if he could no longer do what he did. I wanted to give him something, and I thought the best thing was to ask him to give me something, something of himself. One day, I walked into his room uninvited.

"Mr. Bernanos, you are a priest, is that right?" He nodded, looking up at me expectantly. The lights were off. He kept his room dim, for the light made his headaches worse. His skin was sallow, almost translucent. His face gaunt, his cheeks sunken, with ten days' black whiskers running down to his narrow, sinewy neck—a neck ravaged internally by cancer and surgery. His thin, greasy, uncombed hair, sticking out here and there, was matted to his throbbing head. Perspiration beaded on his taught, unwrinkled forehead, beneath which lurked the unsolved ache. His limbs were frail and thin like an old man's, although he was not yet old. His entire body gave away his fate. Death was coming for him. Yes, death was approaching slowly and painfully.

Why was this man suffering so? Was he a good priest, united to his suffering Lord, crucified on the Cross of his bed in this Calvary of a hospital? Was he a bad priest, and this was his penance for some secret infidelity, some unspeakable sin? Did his suffering have any redemptive value, any purpose? Could any good come from this pain? I could not help but wonder, why did he suffer so?

God's suffering servant Job questioned him, pleading his cause before the divine tribunal. Then, out of the whirlwind, the Lord answered Job. "Who is this that darkens counsel by words without knowledge? Gird up your loins like a man, I will question you, and you shall declare to me. Where were you when I laid the foundation of the earth? Tell me, if you have understanding . . ."[3] Actually, it was not an answer from God to the question of suffering, but a series of questions put to man by God: "I will question you, and you shall declare to me." Whatever answer the infinite God could have provided would no doubt have been beyond Job's finite comprehension.

Likewise, I understood nothing. But as I said, I wanted to give Mr. Bernanos something—or rather, have him give me something of himself, of his purpose. Was this worth anything? We had been taught to always ask patients about their religion or their spirituality: This was a matter of "cultural competence." Polls showed that patients appreciated when doctors prayed with them; so long as it was sincere, this was a good technique for connecting with patients, and so on and so forth. To be honest, I had no interest in any of that—in cultural competence, or technique, or connecting, or advice from those who polled patients.

I knew only this: I wanted to help this man to again be what he once was before the hidden malignant sickness in his head consumed him.

He looked at me, his eyes pools of pain. I asked him, "Could you bless my hands?"

He nodded in assent. Yes.

"Ask God to make them healing hands," I implored.

His dry, colorless lips quivered, almost a smile. I held out my hands, and he took them. Mouthing the words silently, he traced the sign of the cross—the instrument of the God-man's pain—on my palms. I could not hear the words of his silent blessing, could not read his lips, save for the concluding, "In the name of the Father, and of the Son, and of the Holy Spirit." He let go.

"Thank you, father." I nodded, then walked out of the room.

His suffering continued. The days passed. Could I do any more for him? I thought about going into his room to sit with him, perhaps to read him some Psalms. At home, I had even picked out a passage, from Psalm 39:

And now, Lord, for what do I wait? My hope is in thee.

> Deliver me from all my transgressions. Make me not the scorn of the fool.

> I am dumb, I do not open my mouth; for it is thou who hast done it.

> Remove thy stroke from me; I am spent by the blows of thy hand.

> When thou dost chasten man with rebukes for sin, thou dost consume like a moth. What is dear to him; surely every man is a mere breath!

> Hear my prayer, O Lord, and give ear to my cry; hold not thy peace at my tears!

> For I am thy passing guest, a sojourner, like all my fathers.

> Look away from me, that I may know gladness, before I depart and be no more.[4]

But I never again went into his room to read this to him or to keep him company. I made excuses, absurd excuses. Maybe he does not want my company. Maybe he just wants to be left alone. There is no time today. I will do it tomorrow. Tomorrow I will have more time. A few days after asking for his priestly blessing, I came into work resolved to spend a few minutes that day with Father Bernanos, without any more procrastination. As usual, I walked past his room and looked in. The bed was empty. I was too late: He had been transferred to another service. I never saw him again.

He died shortly thereafter. In the quiet of his dark night, death finally came for him. If to suffer most is to be alone, then he died alone—alone with the Alone. Alone with his lonely suffering Lord, who cried out in his last agony, "My God, my God, why have you forsaken me?"

Father Bernanos knew pain. May he rest in peace.

Among all the tissues in the body, when it is irreversibly damaged, the brain alone does not scar. The brain melts. "Liquefactive necrosis" is the medical term for it. Unlike other tissues in the body, the brain does not harden with injury. It liquefies.

"Necrosis," or death of bodily tissue, commonly occurs due to an event doctors call an "infarct." An infarct happens after inadequate oxygen delivery to an organ, resulting in irreversible tissue damage. For example, the medical term for a heart attack is a "myocardial infarct"—the death of heart tissue due to inadequate blood flow, and therefore inadequate oxygen, to the heart muscle. What is commonly called a stroke is in fact an infarct of the brain. After a heart infarct, the heart hardens and scars. After a brain infarct, the brain liquefies and melts.

Mr. Robinson, a fifty-five-year-old gentleman, was sitting on his porch one fine day after work enjoying a beer with his friend.

Something unexpected happened. A tiny plaque broke off the wall of his carotid artery, traveled up the vessels of his neck into the vessels of his head, and lodged itself in the root of the arteries supplying oxygen to the front half of his brain. The blood flow to the frontal lobe of his cerebral cortex immediately ceased. Mr. Robinson collapsed.

The frontal lobe lies at the frontier of modern neuroscience. Its function is largely unknown. The other "lobes" of the brain have been extensively mapped to discrete organic functions; their connections to various other body parts are well elucidated. For example, we know that the back of the brain—the occipital cortex—is responsible for vision and visual processing. We know that the temporal lobes are involved in hearing and memory. The movements of various muscles, the sensations of various regions of the body, have been exhaustively mapped to motor and sensory "strips" near the middle of the cortex. Standard textbooks of neurology contain many diagrams with arrows pointing to various parts of the brain, these parts labeled, their functions explained. But few are the arrows that point to the frontal lobe. In neuroscience, it remains the great unknown.

We know the frontal lobe of humans is larger than that of primates, a fact that has led some scientists to affirm that the frontal lobe is what makes *homo sapiens* unique, what separates humans from other animals. Such metaphysical speculation, although often advanced by scientists, appears to overreach the scientific evidence, which is scant. In what we know of the frontal lobe, which is almost nothing, there is to be found little warrant for this theory. There is a paucity of scientific evidence, and thus, it is an argument from ignorance.

One of the ways neuroscientists have learned the function of various parts of the brain is by observing the loss of function when part of the brain is damaged—for example, by a stroke. There is the famous case of Phineas Gage, a name familiar to every student of neurology. Mr. Gage survived a most astonishing brain injury: After an accidental explosion on the job, a railroad tamping spike went in one side of his head and out the other, impaling large portions of his frontal lobe. The remarkable thing about Phineas Gage, and the reason he is forever inscribed in the annals of medical legend, is that despite the percentage of his brain damaged by the offending spike, he initially appeared to suffer remarkably little motor, sensory, or other neurological dysfunction. It took time for his physicians to realize that he suffered instead from profound changes to his personality.

Mr. Robinson was even less fortunate than the misfortunate Mr. Gage. Mr. Robinson suffered devastating neurological dysfunction. In all the days I observed him, although his muscles were in a state of constant contraction, he never moved. Lying on his bed, his legs were extended railroad-spike straight and scissored together, his right ankle crossed over the left. I reached down to pry them apart but was unable to do so. He was too strong; his contractures would not budge. I managed to squeeze a pillow between his knees. His arms were flexed, also unmoving and unmovable. Awake, his eyes stared into mine. Behind their glassy surface, there appeared to be a distant knowing. It was impossible to tell, however, whether there was any light of conscious awareness left in his mind. I guessed there was, for he always looked as though he wanted to ask something of me. But he could not speak. Another case of quiet desperation.

The brain damage had included dysfunction in "autonomic" centers responsible for involuntary bodily activities like digestion and sweating. How did we know this? The left side of his head was drenched in perspiration, while the right side of his head was bone dry. Down the middle of his face ran a perfectly straight, unmistakable vertical border where sweaty sea met dry desert. The damage to the autonomic center had therefore been unilateral.

"Are you in pain, Mr. Robinson?" I would ask. But it was no use. There was no answer, not a word, not even a look, a turn of the head, a wink, a nod, a wiggling of the finger. Occasionally, he groaned, which is why I suspected he might be in pain. But it was impossible to know for sure. Maybe this was not the groan of a man in physical pain. Maybe it was simply the groan of a man in prison.

One day, a most peculiar thing happened. We were making the daily rounds when we came to Mr. Robinson. We asked the usual perfunctory questions, expecting as usual no intelligible reply. But that day, Mr. Robinson surprised everyone. He turned his head and looked straight at the resident standing next to me. With perfect diction, in a tone so clear that it was unmistakable, he uttered a single word. I should say, rather, he read a single word—read it off of the resident's identification badge hanging on his white coat. Mr. Robinson said, with raised eyebrows and a look of curiosity, "Neurology." Then his face flattened, and his mind receded once again, trailing out of reach. In the days that followed, until the day he was discharged, Mr. Robinson never, to anyone's knowledge, uttered another word.

Neurology. With this one word, Mr. Robinson proved that he could read, he could comprehend, he could speak, he could move. And yet he could not. Or would not? Quiet he remained. Desperate? I think so.

One night, before the "neurology" incident, I was sitting at home after work. My mind drifted to Mr. Robinson. In him, I saw a person with a rigid, mute, half-sweaty body struggling to free himself from invisible chains, from the torture induced by his own liquefying brain. Without understanding why, I was suddenly filled with grief. I wept. Never before in medical school had I cried for a patient, and never since. Which is more perplexing: that I cried for Mr. Robinson, or that I did not cry for the others?

Another question. Which is worse: to suffer, or to watch a loved one suffer?

Mrs. Nantulya had two sons. Both were in the hospital. The four-year-old son was on a respirator in the pediatric intensive care unit. He was suffering from a chronic disease of the lungs. The twenty-year-old son was locked in an isolation room on the psychiatric ward. He was suffering his first schizophrenic break. Mrs. Nantulya divided her time at the hospital between these two sons. She was suffering in the way that only a mother can.

I first saw her with her husband and older son, Yoweri, in the emergency room. Yoweri was having what psychiatrists call a psychotic break, likely his second. At six foot five, he was intimidating. At one point during my interview, he became belligerent and was posturing with an aggressive, threatening stance. The nurse called in security; when they laid hands on him, he fell limp to the ground. His mother stood by, pleading with him to answer my questions. His father sat, staring at the floor, head in his hands, and did not say a word. The family was from Uganda, but all of them spoke English. Clearly, there were cultural barriers to their understanding of Yoweri's mental illness. The parents had brought their son into the hospital after he had tried to open the door and jump out of a moving car. They said he had been acting "funny" for a few weeks.

When addressed, Yoweri stared blankly at me for a few moments, eyelids drooping, mouth closed. Suddenly, he broke into howling laughter, his loud voice startling and unsettling. Then, just as suddenly, the laughter ceased, and his blank stare returned. This was the extent of our communication. The rest of the time, he talked only with the voices, the angels, and God. He claimed to be a prophet. His mother defended this claim. "You would not understand," she told me. "It's a religious thing. He is very religious."

According to his mother, Yoweri's bizarre behavior started two years prior, after he was involved in a car accident. "He hit his head: That's why he acts this way," she insisted. The story alternated between his having prophetic powers and his having a head injury. I suspected a psychotic disorder, a suspicion confirmed a few days later when I checked his old records from a prior psychiatric hospitalization. He had indeed been in a car accident but sustained no head injury. The MRI of his brain was entirely normal. The accident could not account for his psychotic symptoms. His diagnosis: schizophrenia.

Of all chronic illnesses, schizophrenia is perhaps the most devastating. I can think of no other chronic disease that I would less rather have, including Alzheimer's, if only because the latter tends to manifest later in life. To lose one's legs, one's sight, one's hearing—all this is frightening; to lose one's mind is to suffer an even more terrifying indignity. Of all the diagnoses that doctors have to give, schizophrenia is perhaps the most difficult for patients and their families to accept. It breaks into the course of one's life between the ages of fifteen and twenty-five for men, a decade later for women—just when a patient's life as an adult is getting underway. It shatters all of one's plans, projects, and pursuits, replacing them with a life of recurrent hospitalizations, chaotic incoherence, frequent homelessness, and often, a tragic end. Schizophrenia itself is not a fatal illness. However, half of all patients with this diagnosis attempt suicide; ten percent ultimately complete suicide. There is no cure. Current drug treatment is usually burdensome and often not fully effective.

The causes of schizophrenia are unknown; genetics appears to play a significant role, but environmental factors are involved as well. Changes in brain anatomy and neurochemistry have been observed in schizophrenic patients, but the relationships between brain changes and symptoms are not well understood. I tend to think of the symptoms as involving a total disintegration of various mental faculties: Thoughts, sensory perceptions, and emotions become unmoored and fly off, each in their own direction.

For example, schizophrenic patients experience hallucinations—sensory perceptions without external stimuli. These are most frequently auditory (voices "in their head"), often visual (seeing things not really there), sometimes tactile (touch), or rarely olfactory (smell). To the patient, these perceptions seem as vivid as real perceptions; brain imaging studies show that the same areas of the brain are active with hallucinations as are active when the patient is actually seeing or hearing something. This is why hallucinating patients often do things like tear up their walls to find the hidden speaker; this is perfectly rational, given their abnormal perceptions. The voice they hear must be coming from somewhere.

Schizophrenic patients also experience strong delusions—fixed, false, idiosyncratic beliefs, which are not amenable to rational argument. These delusions often exhibit paranoid characteristics, and the patients believe they are being persecuted. The FBI is after me; the aliens are coming to destroy everyone; the doctors are poisoning my food. At other times, the delusions take on grandiose proportions. I am one of the four horsemen of the Apocalypse; I am the Chosen One, destined to bring order out of the chaos; I am a prophet endowed with special powers. I have heard each of these from schizophrenic patients.

These "positive" symptoms—hallucinations and delusions—represent new features of mental life. They are accompanied by "negative" symptoms, which represent deficits in mental life and loss of normal psychological capacities. These can be even more debilitating; they include a total loss of motivation, excessive social withdrawal, attention deficits, and perhaps the most difficult for loved ones, the lack of emotional response or affective warmth. The schizophrenic patient may appear to retreat into an unreal world, no longer able to connect with others in any meaningful way.

It is little wonder that Yoweri's mother refused to accept this diagnosis. His father continued to brood in silence, neither contradicting his wife's insistence that the boy had a head injury or was a prophet, nor agreeing with the doctors that he had a mental illness. Doubtless, they both knew the truth, despite their defensive denials. Their son had been smart, successful in school, and was doing well in college—as is the case for many schizophrenia patients—before his first psychotic break. They could not fathom what had happened to shatter all this.

After we established the diagnosis, the patient and his parents refused continued hospitalization. They chose to let him leave "AMA"—against medical advice—and thus, we could not legally prescribe him medications or set up a follow-up appointment. When we could no longer hold Yoweri against his will, and he was insisting on leaving the psychiatric unit, I went in search of his mother, who I knew was somewhere in the hospital with his brother. I found her in her younger son's pediatric room, watching her little boy's chest rise and fall with the rhythm of the ventilator. Her eyes were swollen and bloodshot. She sat motionless, and moved slowly, exhausted from lack of sleep and emotional anguish.

"Mrs. Nantulya," I said. "Yoweri is leaving. He needs you to take him home." She knew her older son would not be safe on his own, but she did not want to leave her younger son alone. She called her husband.

"He will be here in twenty minutes. Can you keep him until then?" she asked.

"If he insists upon leaving, we cannot legally hold him." The medications had turned down the volume on his hallucinatory voices, but Yoweri was still very delusional, and he ignored most of what we said to him. "We'll do our best to convince him to wait for his father," I told her. She did not respond. "It is important that he follows up with a psychiatrist this week, so that he can get back on medication."

"Yes, I know," she said wearily. She looked defeated. She could not speak it, but she knew the truth, and it was unbearable. Her pain was manifested in a vacant stare, beyond tears. She wavered for a moment. "We will take him to the psychiatrist who treated him after the car accident. He will get treatment."

I hoped that she would follow through.

As a medical student, the experience of seeing so much human suffering was initially jarring, often alarming, and at times dispiriting. I began to wonder whether years of witnessing unrelenting suffering might eventually render me numb to patients' pain, deaf to their cries, blind to their wounds. Would I, with clinical experience, myself become wounded, scarred, even calloused? I did not want to slide down that path, to inadvertently find myself in the blind alley of indifference or ignorance. Although it was a burden, I wanted to keep noticing the quiet desperation behind the eyes of suffering patients and their loved ones. I wanted to keep company with them in their pain.

It is a constant challenge as a physician to navigate this, to avoid becoming calloused or indifferent to human suffering, while not being crushed by it. "The physician comes to know," wrote psychiatrist and philosopher Karl Jaspers in his marvelous essay *The Idea of the Physician*. "He sees the limitations of man, his impotence, his infinite suffering. He sees mental illness, this frightful fact of human existence. He faces death every day."[5] Physicians can never completely rid the world of these afflictions. At times, we can alleviate suffering; always, we can try to act with compassion, to achieve what Jaspers called a "companionship of fate with the sick."[6]

Reflecting on the task of the physician in the face of suffering, Jaspers continued, "It is his nature to show human kindness even where he cannot heal, and to succor even hopeless cases. And as for mental patients, the physician's ethos tells him to furnish these unfortunates, whose health he cannot restore, with a maximum of viability—to honor the human being even in them."[7] Suffering is inseparably bound up with the human condition. For a doctor to ignore or become indifferent to his patients' suffering means that he no longer honors the human being in them. This is what the physician—and the medical student—comes to know.

Medical education and the professional practice of medicine have their pitfalls. My four years in medical school convinced me that doctoring can be dangerous. Jaspers identified three cardinal temptations of doctors—occupational hazards, one could say. "His profession is one of incessant revelations," wrote Jaspers. "The doctor must come to be different from other people. The horrors he sees expose him to great temptations."[8]

First, he may become a skeptic, and later, a cynic, disgusted by all the troubles, frailties, and futilities he has seen. Cynical physicians are on display in Samuel Shem's book *The House of God*, a popular novel about medical interns. The story's amusingly dark humor ultimately degenerates into scornful spite and cynicism. The interns regard most of their patients as "GOMERs" ("get out of my emergency room")—demented elderly who have "lost that which goes into being human." The practice of medicine for these jaded 'terns is a futile system of revolving hospital doors churned by stupid hospital bureaucrats. The disillusioned residents take refuge in orgiastic smut and fantasies of future monetary payoffs for their pointless agonies. The characters in Shem's novel exhibit the folly of succumbing to this first temptation. The cynical physician distorts reality.

The second temptation is toward what Jaspers called "naturalistic fatalism." The physician who gives in to this "sees nothing but causal connections, pitiless nature, and the unexpected turns of chance—the steady flow of coming to be and passing away, in which every individual is a matter of total indifference."[9] For the physician infected by fatalism, patients as unique persons disappear; they are replaced by organs, diseases, and abstractions. Patients are rendered nameless and faceless—"the pancreatitis, the MI, the blue bloater, the pink puffer," and so on.

I remember my irritation at a certain nurse who never bothered to learn her patients' names. One day, when she asked me another question about "twelve," I responded, "What's the patient's name?"

"You know, the patient in room twelve," she said again.

After going back and forth like this a few times, I finally told her, "I don't refer to patients by their room number. Go find out the patient's name and get back to me." My irritation with her was hypocritical, however, for I too had often fallen into similar habits. Doctors must struggle to resist hiding behind the protective veil of lab tests, X-rays, room numbers, and statistics. A physician who succumbs to all this retreats from reality.

The third temptation Jaspers identified is toward nihilism: The physician, he wrote, "may turn into an unbeliever, convinced that there is nothing but this endless cycle of misery. Seeing all the facts that conflict with a harmonious view of the world, he may lose sight of the deity."[10] For doctors, the philosophical problem of evil is not an abstract intellectual riddle, but a daily reality: If the physician cannot find meaning or purpose in the adverse events around him, then he may succumb to atheistic nihilism, denying the world any final meaning or purpose. He may become blinded to the truth that, beyond this vale of tears, the universe has an unshakeable ground of ultimate goodness, which anchors the physician's every act of mercy, lending it eternal weight and meaning. The physician who succumbs to this temptation denies this ultimate reality.

Japsers concludes:

> Skepticism, naturalism, and atheism are the inner perils which may have confronted every physician. It is his way to surmount them which makes for the depth of his vision, for the vigor of his hope, for his passion in spite of everything—the passion of which the poet says, "And by the grave he still unfurls hope's banner." Then he will be undaunted by horror, trusting in an absolute foundation that lends irreplaceable weight to every assistance to men, to each act of love, and to mere human kindness.[11]

There is one final danger that should be mentioned. The physician or medical student may avoid distorting, retreating from, and denying reality, but still succumb to the worst of all temptations. The doctor often sees his fellow man fully unveiled in all his naked vulnerability, his tragic frailty and folly. Seeing his neighbor in all his nakedness may lead the physician to despise him, and to develop what Jaspers called a ruinous sense of one's own superiority. To set himself above his patients is perhaps the worst error a doctor can make. I have seen medical students, residents, and attendings fall prey to this hubris. I am far from immune myself. The temptation to pride is perhaps the most difficult for a physician to surmount.

Given the powers that society and technology place in his hands, modesty does not always come easily for a doctor. The medical profession has been plagued, probably since the days of Hippocrates, with the stereotype of the arrogant physician who thinks he is a god. It is an image we would do well to shed. Socrates claimed that he was the only wise man in Athens, because he realized that he was the only one who knew that he was not yet wise.

For those students who are willing to learn the lesson, who are attentive to the realities that surround them, medical school is a school of humility, sometimes humiliation, because one learns very quickly how little one knows. The perceptive medical student will realize that any pride in this game is both false and foolish. What T. S. Eliot wrote about life generally can be applied to the experienced physician: "The only wisdom we can hope to acquire is the wisdom of humility."[12]

Even—perhaps especially—when one has finished medical school, one's ignorance can seem daunting. But awareness of this is a good thing, not a shortcoming. Doctors who have acquired the wisdom of humility are no longer afraid to answer patients' intractable questions by simply admitting, "I don't know." For if those doctors have real compassion, if they are willing to suffer just a bit with their patients, physicians need not have all the answers.

CHAPTER 10

Diagnosing the Disease

Listen to your patient, he is telling you the diagnosis.
—Sir William Osler[1]

A few short years after completing the arduous process of acceptance into medical school, the task of applying to residency programs began. Once again, we collected letters of recommendation, we agonized over personal statements, we traveled all over the country to interview at various programs. All this happened during the fourth and final year of med school. Although clinical duties lightened, we still struggled to fit travel time into a busy schedule of rotations. Life in medical school never really slowed down.

There is one key difference between acceptance into residency programs and acceptance into college or medical school. With the latter, if the applicant is a strong candidate, he receives acceptance letters from multiple schools; then the applicant chooses among programs where he got in. Residency is different: There is no choice among programs that one gets into. Rather, the applicant "matches" to a single program, and that is the end of it.

This is roughly how the match works: The applicant "ranks" the programs where he interviewed in the order of his preference. He is free to rank as few or as many programs as he wishes. The programs, in turn, also rank all the students who interviewed with them. Then a unique pairing process takes place, an event that is probably without parallel for its scope, complexity, and impact on so many individuals. On midnight, a week or so before Match Day, a mysterious and powerful computer-in-the-cloud—call him Zeus—runs a complicated algorithm, which only a handful of MIT graduates are capable of understanding. By means of this program, Zeus decides the fate of nearly forty thousand senior medical students. This potent supercomputer matches every applicant to a single residency program. This is his or her fate. End of discussion.

I stared down at the white envelope in my hand. Sealed inside was a slip of paper on which was written my destination for the next four years. The previous four years seemed to focus, to concentrate on the residency program named inside the white envelope.

I looked up. My wife stood next to me, our son in her arms. I glanced around. The rest of the auditorium was filled with my classmates, each of whom also held in hand his or her own white envelope—their own sealed fate. Parents had driven or flown long distances to be here; spouses had taken the day off work; siblings had skipped school to attend. This was March 20—known at every medical school around the nation as Match Day.

Across the US, every fourth-year medical student was also standing, at precisely that moment, holding a white envelope. The various medical schools had all adjusted for time zone differences, so that the East Coast students would not discover before the West Coast students where they had matched. In all fifty states, every senior med student would open his envelope simultaneously.

"No peeking," said our dean from the podium. He grinned. "It's almost time."

Here we stood, holding the prize or punishment that Zeus had dealt us. Our dean leaned over the microphone and began the countdown. "Ten, nine, eight, seven," we joined in the counting, "six, five, four, three . . ." My hand trembled slightly as I peeled open the envelope. The page was blank . . . no, wait . . . turn it over . . . now there is too much writing . . . where is the important part? Where is the . . . ah, yes. UC Irvine, my first choice. California, here we come! My wife hugged me. Dr. Burke, my resident mentor who was standing behind me, congratulated me. Our son John, still in Jennifer's arms, looked around in bewilderment, wondering what all the commotion was about. The classmate next to me embraced her mother, both crying happy tears. Others left the room quickly, trying to conceal their disappointment. It was quite a scene that fateful day, there in the usually placid lecture auditorium. I was grateful to be among those who stuck around afterward to celebrate.

Nevertheless, there was a bittersweet side to that day as well. I expected this, regardless of the match outcome. Jennifer and I had decided, after living away from both our families for four difficult years, it was time to move back west. Especially now that we had a child, we wanted John to grow up near his extended family and have the support of relatives nearby during my residency. Unfortunately, her family was in California and mine in Washington State. We could not live near both families. Therefore, I let the residency program be the deciding factor in my rankings between the two. Both were great programs, but in the end, the California program was a better fit than the Washington program. I knew that either way, one side of the family would naturally be disappointed, although both would understand. The phone call to my parents would not be easy. I give them credit for their unwavering love and support.

It is often the choices between competing goods—the choices that look like a no-lose situation—that prove to be the most difficult. At times, I would prefer it if someone else chose for me. I was thankful, therefore, that this decision was not entirely within my power. For me, there was only the ranking. The rest was not my business.

While I have never regretted my decision to become a doctor, I am chagrined to report that the realities on the ground in contemporary medicine often contrast with the hopeful joys and optimism of Match Day, when I set off on my career path as a physician.

First, patients seem unhappy with the state of contemporary medicine. Aspects of this dissatisfaction include, among other problems, poor communication, long wait times, high costs, barriers to access, and a perceived lack of respect or trust in the healthcare system. According to Pew Research Center, the number of US adults who place confidence in medical scientists to act in the best interests of the public declined from 40 percent in 2020 to 29 percent in 2022.[2] A 2021 survey by the American Board of Internal Medicine likewise found that one in six people—including physicians—no longer trust doctors, and one in three do not trust the healthcare system. Likewise, almost half the population does not trust our public health agencies to act in our interests.[3]

These numbers worsened after institutional medicine's serious failures and its slide into authoritarianism during the Covid crisis—themes I explored in my book *The New Abnormal: The Rise of the Biomedical Security State*.[4] A 2022 survey reported that 60 percent of Americans had a negative healthcare experience in the prior three months, with just 40 percent rating US healthcare quality as "very good" or "good"—a significant drop from earlier highs. In this study, half of those with declining trust in healthcare pointed to self-interested motives over patient care.[5] Similarly, a 2023 poll commissioned by the American Academy of Physician Associates found that over 70 percent of US adults believe the healthcare system fails them, while half of Americans surveyed reported their symptoms were "ignored, dismissed, or not believed" by providers.[6] A 2020 study published in the *Journal of the American Medical Association* found one in five adults experienced discrimination in healthcare, often repeatedly, eroding trust and satisfaction.[7]

Patients are not the only ones dissatisfied with the current state of institutional medicine. As I also mentioned in the introduction, doctors are leaving the profession in droves, prompting worries of a worsening physician shortage. Why is medicine today failing many of its brightest students and pushing large numbers of its seasoned practitioners into early retirement? The answer is complex and multifactorial, but a major contributing factor is the managerial revolution in medicine.

Medicine, like many other contemporary institutions since World War II, has succumbed to managerialism—the unfounded belief that everything can and should be deliberately engineered and managed from the top down by a cadre of supposed experts. Managerialism is destroying good medicine.

The managerialist ideology consists of several core tenets, as outlined by N. S. Lyons.[8] The first is Technocratic Scientism, or the belief that everything, including society and human nature, can and should be fully understood and controlled through materialist scientific and technical means, and that those with superior scientific and technical knowledge are therefore best placed to govern society. In medicine, this manifests through the metastatic proliferation of top-down "guidelines" that are imposed on physicians to dictate the management of various illnesses. These come not just from professional medical societies, but also from state and federal regulatory authorities and public health agencies.

"Guidelines" is, in fact, a euphemism designed to obscure their actual function: They control a physician's behavior by dictating payments and reimbursement for hitting certain metrics. In 1990, the number of available guidelines was 70; by 2012, there were over 7,500. In this metastatic managerialist regime, the physician's clinical discretion goes out the window, sacrificed on the altar of unthinking checklists. If the case histories recounted in this book have conveyed nothing else, hopefully they at least convinced the reader that every patient is *sui generis*, unrepeatably unique. One cannot practice good medicine with a one-size-fits-all cookbook.

Real patients, in their unique individuality, cannot be adequately managed with a diagnostic-based algorithm or treated by an iPad. At best, checklists are useful only once the problem has been thoroughly understood. For the practitioner to be able to make sense of problems in the first place requires intuition and imagination—both attributes in which humans will always have the edge over the computer. Problem-solving in a complex environment involves cognitive processes analogous to creative endeavors, but medical education as currently configured does not cultivate in students these imaginative capacities.[9]

Technocratic Scientism has likewise driven the campaign for so-called "evidence-based medicine"—the application of rationalized expert knowledge, gleaned typically from controlled trials, to individual clinical cases. At first glance, the idea of evidence-based medicine seems hard to argue with—after all, shouldn't medical interventions be based on the best available evidence? But there are serious flaws with this model, which have been exploited by big pharma. Studies yield statistical averages, which apply to populations but say nothing about individuals. No two human bodies are exactly alike; but Technocratic Scientism treats bodies as fungible and interchangeable.

As my colleague Yale epidemiologist Harvey Risch has argued, "evidence-based medicine" (EBM)—a term coined by Gordon Guyatt in 1990—sounds plausible but is really a sham.[10] Of course, physicians have been reasoning from empirical evidence since ancient times; to suggest otherwise only betrays ignorance of the history of medicine. EBM proponents claim we should only use the "best available evidence" to make clinical judgments. But this sleight-of-hand is deceptive and wrongheaded: We should use *all* available evidence, not just that deemed "best" by self-appointed "experts." The term "evidence-based" functions to smuggle in the claim that blinded, randomized, placebo-controlled trials (RCTs) are always the best form of evidence, and therefore the gold standard for medical knowledge.

But as Risch explains, "Judgments about what constitutes 'best' evidence are highly subjective and do not necessarily yield overall results that are quantitatively the most accurate and precise."[11] Every study design has its own strengths and weaknesses, including RCTs. Randomization is only one among many methods in research study design for controlling potential confounding factors, and it only works if you end up with large numbers of subjects in the relevant outcome arm. The EBM model unjustifiably favors randomized controlled trials that only large pharmaceutical companies can afford to conduct to license their products.

This results in, among other things, the scrapping of the entire discipline of epidemiology, which relies on study methods other than RCTs. "Evidence-based medicine's" criteria constitute big pharma propaganda masquerading as the "best" expert scientific and technical knowledge. In Risch's words, "Representing that only highly unaffordable RCT evidence is appropriate for regulatory approvals provides a tool for pharma companies to protect their expensive, highly profitable patent products against competition by effective and inexpensive off-label approved generic medications whose manufacturers would not be able to afford large-scale RCTs."[12] Moneyed interests, not scientific methodology, drive so-called evidence-based medicine.

The second tenet of the managerialist ideology is Utopian Progressivism, or the belief that a perfect society is possible through precise application of scientific and technical knowledge, and that the Arc of History bends towards utopia as more expert knowledge is acquired. I recall a conversation a few years ago with a nurse ethicist from Johns Hopkins who was giving a guest lecture at the medical school where I taught. She remarked that Johns Hopkins Hospital deployed the marketing tagline "The Place Where Miracles Happen." Medicine is clearly not immune from Utopian Progressivism, even if it's only cynically tapping into this ideology for public relations and advertising purposes.

Naturally, promising to deliver miracles only sets up physicians for failure and patients for disappointment. When those promised miracles fail to materialize—an incurable cancer is every bit as incurable at Hopkins as it was at your local community hospital—patients feel betrayed and doctors bereft. A humble and realistic acknowledgment of the permanent limits of medicine is a necessary starting point for any sane and sustainable healthcare system. Doctors are not miracle-workers, much less gods. Science cannot save us.

The third feature of the managerialist ideology is Liberationism, the belief that individuals and societies are held back from progress by the rules, restraints, relationships, historical institutions, communities, and traditions of the past—all of which are necessarily inferior to the new, and which we must therefore be liberated from in order to move forward. Contrary to this ideology, there are some things in medicine that will never change. As I argued in chapter 7, at its foundation, medicine is constituted by a particular kind of relationship—a relationship based upon trust between a patient made vulnerable by illness and a doctor who professes to use his knowledge and skills always and only for the purposes of health and healing. No technological advance and no societal development will ever alter this. The ends or purposes of medicine are baked into the kind of profession that it is, grounded in the permanent realities of health, illness, and the human body.

But today, the ideology of Liberationism seeks to "free" medicine from these constraints. Why should physicians only pursue health and healing among their goals? After all, biomedical technology can be used for all kinds of other ends. In addition to making the sick well, we can make the healthy "better than well": Through hormones, gene editing, or psychopharmacology, we can make short people tall, weak people strong, and average people more intelligent. These projects of "human enhancement" will explode the boundaries of medicine and liberate man from the constraints of human nature. Why limit ourselves to healing when we can turn men into women, women into men, and humans into bigger, faster, stronger, smarter superhumans or post-humans? Liberationist projects promise to free man not just from the ravages of illness, but from the constraints of human nature itself.

A thorough critique of projects of so-called human enhancement would require a separate book. Suffice it to say that our early forays into these domains have proven to be not liberating but dehumanizing. To take just one contemporary example, what proponents call "gender affirmative care" is quickly crumbling under the weight of evidence showing that puberty-blocking hormones, cross-sex hormones, and surgeries that destroy healthy reproductive organs have not improved the mental health outcomes of gender dysphoric youth. The United Kingdom and various Scandinavian countries, which have commissioned reports to carefully examine the scientific evidence for these interventions, are quickly shuttering their pediatric gender clinics before additional harm is inflicted on vulnerable young people struggling with body image and identity issues.[13]

However, we did not need this scientific evidence—helpful as it is to make the case—to understand that destroying the function of healthy organs is not a good idea. How could this entire enterprise possibly be compatible with good medicine, with the goals of health and human flourishing internal to the practice of medicine? What has unfolded in the last several years with the explosion of gender affirmative care was largely driven not just by the Liberationist ideology, but also by financial considerations and the desire to create a cohort of lifelong patients, entirely dependent on the healthcare system, who otherwise were physically healthy. The result has been a form of institutionalized and medicalized child abuse fueled by social contagion and sustained by the slander and silencing of critics. Gender medicine is poised to soon globally collapse under the weight of its own contradictions and will be remembered as one of the greatest scandals and follies of medical history.

The fourth feature of the managerial revolution is Homogenizing Universalism, or the belief that all human beings are fundamentally interchangeable units of a single universal group, and that the systemic "best practices" discovered by scientific management are universally applicable in all places and for all peoples. Therefore, any non-superficial particularity or diversity of place, culture, custom, nation, or government structure anywhere is evidence of an inefficient failure to converge successfully on the ideal system. According to this tenet, progress always naturally entails centralization and homogenization.

As with the "clinical guidelines" discussed above, medicine has also seen the recent explosion of so-called quality metrics for medical providers and organizations. These drive homogenizing universalism in medicine, which dictates that every patient gets the same cookie-cutter care. For example, a 2020 study published in *JAMA* found that the Centers for Medicare and Medicaid Services had over 2,200 quality measures in its inventory, with approximately 800 in use, reflecting an explosion in these measurement efforts over time.[14] This does not include the additional metrics from private insurers, state programs, and other organizations. These measures, numbering in the thousands, cost each physician at least $40,000 annually to manage, translating to roughly $15.4 billion nationwide—costs that get passed on to patients.[15]

There is no substantial evidence that these improve medical outcomes. In fact, this Homogenizing Universalism often worsens medical results by mandating a one-size-fits-all approach to clinical care. This compromises physicians' appropriate clinical judgment and necessary discretionary latitude. Doctors are pushed to hit metrics on measurements like blood pressure, even if this does not actually improve meaningful outcomes like heart attacks or strokes. These guidelines are often pushed by industry groups who have a vested interest in expanding disease categories or widening disease definitions. "Let's lower the threshold for what counts as hypertension or high cholesterol, so more patients get on antihypertensives and statins," for example. If doctors don't comply, they don't get paid. It does not matter whether placing more patients on statins fails to save lives.[16]

This leads, among other issues, to "preventative" overprescribing. In the US, 25 percent of people in their 60s are on five or more long-term medications, rising to 46 percent of people in their 70s and 91 percent of nursing home residents. The evidence supporting the use of these drugs is based on younger, healthier people. Nursing home residents are generally excluded from clinical trials of new medications. And yet the norm for elderly adults is a multi-drug regimen, often for the theoretical prevention of future outcomes rather than the measurable treatment of existing disease. Calling this "evidence-based medicine" strains credulity. It is pharma-driven, profit-driven interventionism. We often have too much, not too little, medicine.

This is an old story. In his classic book *The Canterbury Tales*, the fourteenth-century poet Geoffrey Chaucer satirized physicians: "For gold in phisik [medicine] is a cordial, / Therefore he [the physician] lovede gold in special." Chaucer here puns on "cordial" (a healing tonic), suggesting the physician loves money more than healing, and implying his treatments prolong illness for profit. Chaucer also notes the physician's "special love" for the apothecary, hinting at a shady partnership where doctors and druggists overprescribe for mutual gain—a critique of medieval physicians still resonant today.[17]

We see evidence of Homogenizing Universalism everywhere now in medical institutions that function according to the principle of efficient people-moving—what I call "turnstile" medicine. In this system, patients themselves become the manufactured products of our standardized, industrialized healthcare system.[18] Medicare's bundled payments under the Affordable Care Act treat every hip-replacement the same, incentivizing hospital administrators to focus on "throughput"—moving patients through the system as quickly as possible. A patient who takes a bit longer to recover from surgery or develops a complication becomes a financial liability for the hospital. This statistical outlier is resented for not behaving according to the principles of maximum efficiency and patient uniformity.

To mention another example, while I understand it's a quality control measure designed to reduce medication errors, hospitals now scanning the barcode on the patient's wristband to verify the correct medical record or medication turns patients into supermarket items or cattle. We should not ignore the symbolic effects of our practices on actual human beings. Depersonalized managerialist medicine is no replacement for doctors and nurses who know their patients personally and can therefore verify they are looking at the right chart or administering the correct medication.

Excessive centralized administrative control is not a sign of institutional vigor but is evident in the decline of every civilization. Bloated bureaucracies grow rigid, corrupt, and increasingly detached from the realities they are supposed to govern. Overreach stifles innovation, while rigid controls impede adaptability, and mismanagement bleeds resources. By the third century AD, Rome's sprawling empire leaned on a bloated and increasingly inefficient bureaucracy.[19] The Han Dynasty in China, which crumbled also in the third century AD, showed a similar pattern of top-heavy administrative rot.[20] Likewise with the Maya city-states around 900 AD, where overzealous elites exercising centralized control ignored the real problems on the ground in favor of their pet projects and preoccupations.[21] The centralized administrative control characteristic of managerialism threatens institutional medicine in the same ways today.

What primarily ails medicine is not just technical problems or economic challenges, important as these issues are to address. Our deepest problems are philosophical, fueled by ideologies that distort the nature and purpose of medicine. The iron cage created by this system appears difficult to break free from. The only solution, I believe, is the development of parallel medical institutions—entirely new models of clinical care and reimbursement—started by physicians that opt out of this perverse system entirely. I will explore this further in the next chapter. It will take imaginative minds to establish such a system, but the demand is present if we can create the supply. Creative doctors are already at work developing models of subscription-based direct primary care and other parallel medical systems.

Medicine has always been hierarchical, but never has it been so conformist—with too many uncritical, thoughtless physicians marching in lockstep to hit metrics dictated by vested outside interests that show little concern for sick patients. Will we recognize that the managerialist ideology undermines medicine's goals of health and summon the will necessary to slice through all obstacles and eliminate the excrescences that undermine the ability of physicians to heal? Will we, in short, make the cut?

Contrary to the myth of automatic progress in society or in science, for any culture or profession, knowledge once gained can be lost. There is a real danger that we will squander the art of medicine, forgetting things we once knew and failing to pass them on to the next generation of physicians. To take one simple example, the careful medical history and skilled physical examination—the mainstay of the physician's diagnostic repertoire—are now mostly replaced with indiscriminate batteries of expensive and time-consuming tests and imaging procedures.

We favor the high-tech scanner over the low-tech stethoscope. We rush through the history to get to the lab tests. But these scans and tests are worse than useless if we do not know what we are looking for. Ninety percent of good diagnostics come from the history, from talking patiently and listening carefully to the patient, and from meticulous observation. For a skilled physician, diagnostic tests typically confirm what we already know. And if we don't know much before ordering a battery of tests, they will do more harm than good, sending us down rabbit holes to work up incidental or meaningless findings or anomalies, which invariably turn up with excessive testing or imaging.

I will be the first to celebrate novel medical technologies that improve patient outcomes and help doctors to save lives. I am a fan of science and technology. But scientific advances and technological innovations alone will not save medicine. Whether the influence of big pharma that profits from sickness, compromised public health agencies captured and controlled by the very industries they are supposed to regulate, a biosecurity state that tends to jump from one declared health emergency to the next, or the current replication crisis in biomedical research where study findings routinely fail to be replicated by other researchers,[22] medicine is now in danger of causing more sickness than it heals.

Fifty years ago, Ivan Illich's prophetic book *Medical Nemesis* opened with the startling claim, "The medical establishment has become a major threat to health."[23] The book explores the epidemic of iatrogenic disease—that is, illnesses caused by medical interventions—which has only worsened in the nearly half century since its publication. Most of the current research literature on iatrogenesis focuses on the problem of medical errors and how to institute systems that can minimize errors. This is obviously important, but medical errors are only part of the story of how medicine is harming us.

Illich's thesis is that some systems, including our healthcare system, improve outcomes only until they expand to a certain industrialized size, monopolistic scope, and level of technological power. Once this threshold is surpassed, without intending to do so, these systems paradoxically cannot help but inflict harm and undermine their stated aims. Illich diagnosed "the disease of medical progress" in its early stages; I believe that almost half a century later, this disease has now reached its advanced stage.

The problem is political and not merely professional: "the layman and not the physician has the potential perspective and effective power to stop the current iatrogenic epidemic."[24] Indeed, "among all our contemporary experts, physicians are those trained to the highest level of specialized incompetence for this urgently needed pursuit."[25] Physicians are too embedded in the pathogenic system to offer the cure. The solution must be primarily patient-driven.

Organized medicine has always carefully guarded its membership and monopoly on professional privileges, from ordering tests to prescribing medications. This medical monopolistic control has expanded without checks and has encroached on our liberties regarding our own bodily integrity and our common life together in community.[26] In my previous book, *The New Abnormal*, I explored how this tendency manifested during our disastrous response to Covid. But the problem is not limited to that period of recent medical history; the destructive public health response to Covid was merely a symptom of more widespread problems in our healthcare system.

As described in the previous section, the failed reaction to medicine's ills so far has been more managerialism—more top-down control by so-called "experts"—but this has only worsened the crisis. Similarly, simple demands for the delivery of more medical care will, paradoxically, only exacerbate the problem. "The self-medication of the medical system cannot but fail," as Illich put it.[27] You cannot solve a problem using the very same means that created the problem in the first place.

A professionalized, physician-driven system of healthcare that expands beyond its critical limit exacerbates illness for three reasons. First, an overly expansive healthcare system will tend to inflict clinical damage that eventually outweighs health benefits. Second, the system tends to worsen the social conditions that render society unhealthy. Third, it tends to expropriate the power of the individual to heal himself, placing that power exclusively in the hands of professionalized experts. The solution therefore must involve a political program that facilitates the reappropriation of personal responsibility for healthcare, combined with sensible limits to the professional management of our health. In short: To save medicine, we must limit medicine. Paradoxically, the cure for our epidemic of ill health will require less, not more, professionalized healthcare.

Medicine has developed powerful, self-serving myths to hide these inconvenient truths. Modern medicine has long exaggerated its effectiveness, though these myths have been documented and debunked by historians of medicine and public health. A few examples here will suffice, though these could be multiplied. Although we can now treat it with antibiotics, medicine did not cure tuberculosis: In New York in 1812, the death rate was 700 per 10,000; by the time the offending bacillus was isolated in 1882, but before treatment was available, the death rate was nearly half that at 370 per 10,000. In 1910 when the first sanitarium was opened, the death rate had declined to 180. Following World War II, but before antibiotics for tuberculosis were developed, it had plummeted to 48.[28] Medicine was clearly not responsible for the cure, which came about through improved hygiene and better social conditions.

Other infectious diseases of the last hundred years—from cholera, dysentery, and typhoid to diphtheria, measles, and scarlet fever—likewise peaked and declined apart from and prior to vaunted medical therapies like antibiotics or vaccines.[29] This decline was due primarily to improved host resistance from better nutrition, and secondarily to improvements in housing, sanitation, and other living conditions. "Food, water, and air, in correlation with the level of sociopolitical equality and the cultural mechanisms that make it possible to keep the population stable, play the decisive role in determining how healthy grown-ups feel and at what age adults tend to die."[30] In other words, progress against these infectious diseases came from the main tools of the original Hippocratic physicians, who focused primarily on dietetics and environment and only secondarily on drugs and surgery.

As Illich summarized, "The professional practice of physicians cannot be credited with the elimination of old forms of mortality or morbidity, nor should it be blamed for the increased expectancy of life spent in suffering from the new diseases."[31] Instead, undernourishment in poor countries and poisons and mutagens in our ultra-processed food and the environment in rich nations are the major factors contributing to our current epidemic of chronic illness today. Ozempic for everyone cannot cure our metabolic woes.

The epidemic of iatrogenic disease can no longer be hidden. People are waking up to realize that power over their health has been taken from them.[32] They want to reappropriate what they have relinquished to an ineffective healthcare system that no longer serves their needs. It is increasingly apparent that modern medicine now frequently serves industrial, not personal, growth. Its highest aim is not health but efficiency. "Throughput" is a favorite buzzword of hospital administrators, who copy the people-moving engineering of Disneyland to create turnstile systems that shuffle people through the medical machinery without resolving their issues. Hospitals and clinics have become factories with processed patients as the product.

The practice of medicine is now about efficiently and predictably controlling bodies more than healing them. In the process, physicians have become glorified data-gathering clerks, staring at a computer screen in the consulting room rather than engaging in face-to-face dialogue with the patient. Doctors ask a series of questions dictated by external managers that have little or nothing to do with the patient's chief complaint. Patients leave these encounters feeling bewildered, unheard, unhelped, and unhealed.

Following the managerialist revolution in medicine, even medical harms are depersonalized and dismissed as minor glitches in otherwise functional medical machinery. While doctor-inflicted pain and injury have always been a risk of medical interventions, "With the transformation of the doctor from an artisan exercising a skill on personally known individuals into a technician applying scientific rules to classes of patients, malpractice acquired an anonymous, almost respectable status," as Illich describes. "What had formerly been considered an abuse of confidence and a moral fault can now be rationalized into the occasional breakdown of equipment and operators."[33] Even medical errors take on an anonymous, depersonalized tone in a managerialist system. Nobody is really responsible when things go sideways.

These harms cannot be reversed by more technical or managerial measures—which will only exacerbate the problems they created in the first place by a self-reinforcing feedback loop. Health is not a commodity that can be mass-produced on an engineering model. As Illich explained, "The more time, toil, and sacrifice spent by a population in producing medicine as a commodity, the larger will be the by-product, namely, the fallacy that society has a supply of *health* locked away which can be mined and marketed."[34] The solution can only come from individuals re-appropriating responsibility for their health, and thereby limiting the expansive industrial scope of medical systems. Just to mention one offhand example, perhaps we should abolish the "note from the doctor." Why should physicians exercise a monopoly on declaring someone sick? Why should suffering, mourning, or healing outside the medically designated patient role be considered a form of social deviance?

Without doubt, a limited number of medical procedures and a handful of medications (perhaps a few dozen time-tested drugs) have proven extremely useful. For example, antibiotics for pneumonia, syphilis, malaria, and other serious infectious diseases are effective when used judiciously to avoid breeding drug resistant bugs. Medicine has its tools, and we sometimes need them. It's telling, however, that pharmaceutical companies invest almost nothing in research and development for new antibiotics, because a one-time prescription drug that cures a problem is not sufficiently profitable.[35]

Companies instead want drugs for chronic conditions that can be mitigated but not cured by medications; they want meds that you must take forever. However, the effectiveness of medications for chronic, non-infectious diseases has been much less impressive. Some cancer screenings and therapies have improved survival outcomes, but cancer rates continue to rise due to environmental and lifestyle factors, including among young adults.[36] Psychiatric medications can be lifesaving but are frequently overprescribed and often misused.[37] Medications alone are not the answer to our chronic disease epidemic.

We need to explore how some of our best medical tools can be de-professionalized. Some of the most effective drugs, for example, are sufficiently safe that they could be made available over the counter or following a simple screening for drug allergies or obvious contraindications. Organized medicine and medical societies, including the AMA, have strenuously resisted such proposals, since these organizations exist to lobby for the maintenance of medical monopolies and the pecuniary interests of physicians. Our massive investment in medicine—we spend twice as much of our GDP on healthcare as any other nation and get worse outcomes than most developed countries[38]—is enriching specialist physicians but clearly not improving health outcomes.

Among high-income countries, the US has the lowest life expectancy, the highest rates of avoidable deaths, the highest maternal and infant mortality, the highest rate of people with multiple chronic conditions, an obesity rate nearly twice the average of other developed nations, and among the highest suicide rates.[39] If monopolistic medicine has failed to deliver the goods, then it is time to break up this monopoly. The necessary "surgery" for our healthcare system will be painful for some and will encounter strong resistance from entrenched interests. But it's time for us to make the cut.

Our costly medical bureaucracies stress the delivery of repair and maintenance services for human bodies broken by modern social systems: Too many people have been reduced to the human components of our societal megamachine.[40] Physicians become auto mechanics for cars whose engines are forced to chronically redline, relentlessly pushed beyond their engineered limits. We doctors are told to open the hood and fix them, to get these cars—these broken-down bodies—back on a racetrack they were never designed to drive on. More equitable delivery of medical repair and maintenance services will not resolve the underlying problems: The current system is set up to fail.

Medical care has been massively centralized, even in healthcare systems like the US has that are neither nationalized nor based upon a single government payer. The only way out of this dead-end aporia is decentralization. We must give people back sovereignty and responsibility for their own health and provide them with the means to access healthcare that does not rely entirely on medical gatekeepers. I appreciate MRIs every bit as much as the next doctor, but universally available vitamin D would do more for the nation's health than all our expensive imaging scanners at a fraction of the cost.

In contrast to our reigning model of top-down technocratic medicine, which attempts to manipulate masses of passive bodies into a state of health, traditional Hippocratic medicine sees the individual dynamic human body as the primary agent of health and healing. On this view, the body is an integrated, organic whole, naturally oriented to health and human flourishing. However, the body encounters threats and obstacles to the realization of these ends in the form of disease and injury. Medicine's primary role is to remove these obstacles so that the body can heal itself.

A surgeon does not really "close" a surgical wound; she merely positions the tissues together with sutures so that the body can heal the wound itself. Since it is naturally oriented toward health and wholeness, the body does most of the work. Similarly, antibiotics alone do not rid the body of infections: They merely lower the infectious load sufficiently to allow the body's own immune system to eradicate the pathogen. For this reason, antibiotics are of no avail in a patient who is too severely immunocompromised, as happens in advanced AIDS, for example. Again, the body is the primary agent of healing. Good medicine works with the body as its assistant, in a subordinate role. Nature is the norm of health for Hippocratic medicine.

By contrast, contemporary medicine is undergirded by the mechanistic-technocratic ideology of scientism—the (nonscientific) ideology that science is the only valid form of knowledge. In this view, there is no such thing as human nature, defined by the well-working of an organic body with its own intrinsic ends. The body is reduced to dumb matter, inert purposeless raw material that might just as well be dead as alive. For the technocratic mindset, the reference point for medicine is no longer the healthy human body as an integrated whole, which needs to be supported and maintained by working with the body's own innate capacities. As I suggested in the discussion of cadaver dissection in chapter 2, the reference point for modern medicine is literally the corpse—or at least the sick body—which needs to be technologically vivified and periodically updated from the outside.

On this conception, the human body has no holistic form in itself: It is merely a grab-bag of discreet physiological functions, each of which can be externally commandeered and reconfigured. This false account of human life drives much of the sick-making machinery of modern medicine. Authentic reform will require recovering a Hippocratic philosophy in which medicine serves as the body's apprentice instead of its master. Medicine's relationship to the body should be one of humble assistance, not of overweening power.

Healthcare is primarily something one does, not something one markets or buys. Health can be cultivated but cannot be purchased. But our current system trains us for healthcare *consumption* rather than for health promoting *action*; indeed, the healthcare system itself constrains our range of autonomous action. Remedies available only by prescription become for many virtually unobtainable for patients and families accustomed in past generations to caring for themselves and their loved ones.

Most strategies for medical reform will fail because they focus too much on sickness and too little on changing the environment—the over-processed food, the environmental toxins, the stress-inducing demands of advanced industrialized societies—that makes people sick in the first place. Public health must attend to these serious problems. However, the cure is neither more environmental engineering nor more human engineering efforts to adapt people to a disease-inducing environment. For humans are not designed to be cogs in an engineered machine.

The problems of overly industrialized medicine will not be solved by industrialized and professionalized public health. Instead, according to Illich, "The [real] level of public health corresponds to the degree to which the means and responsibility for coping with illness are distributed among the total population," not monopolized by an elite class of supposed "experts."[41] Good medical intervention can enhance but never replace our acquired ability to cope with illness or disability. Modest public health measures can remove some of the obstacles to health and human flourishing if kept within due limits. Reducing professional intervention to a minimum need not deprive us of necessary help; these limits can aid in health-promoting cultural conditions and practices. For, as Illich writes in pointing out an obvious truth we are inclined to forget, "Healthy people need minimal bureaucratic interference to mate, give birth, share the human condition, and die."[42]

Further increases in medical controls are not the answer to our ills, for this will only worsen iatrogenic harms. We cannot allow the whole world to become one vast hospital—a recipe not for health but for a dystopian totalitarian system run by an elite cadre of physician-therapists in white coats, where anesthetized patients become solitary, passive, and impotent. Many patients today, sadly, already experience this state of helpless unfreedom—what Illich calls "compulsory survival in a planned and engineered hell"[43]—where our sickness only grows worse. The solution to our health woes will require empowering individuals and small communities with the tools necessary not only to heal, but also to cope with the inevitabilities of pain, impairment, and eventual death. Dependence on, and addiction to, a malignant managerialized system will only make us sicker.

Contrary to our technocratic fever-dreams, human nature is not infinitely elastic, but has inherent limits that medicine will never overcome, however powerful our technical tools become. Consistent with such limits, it is time for us to develop decentralized, small-scale initiatives that operate autonomously, apart from the managerialized systems of medical power. Self-healing is possible just as self-education is possible, without entirely discarding the undeniable benefits of larger-scale organized medicine or educational institutions—so long as these are kept within reasonable limits.

As the Ancient Greek tragedians knew, hubris brings downfall. Try to construct a Tower of Babel and it will eventually collapse. Any medicine that does not embrace rational restraint—that does not make the necessary cuts—will end up inflicting more harm than healing. It's time to recall that health is mostly something one *does* in the context of a supportive family and community, more than something one is *granted* from external agents or professional experts. Physicians, and the associated technologies of modern medicine, can play a supportive role in a sane and humane healthcare system, but we are not the lead actors in the drama of health and human flourishing.

CHAPTER 11

Making the Cut

There are in truth no specialties in medicine, since to know fully many of the most important diseases a man must be familiar with their manifestations in many organs.
—Sir William Osler[1]

It saddens me to report, as we explored in the previous chapter, that our medical institutions—from hospitals and licensing boards to medical schools and professional societies—are failing us. The complex of problems in many of these institutions makes reform or repair, in the short term at least, impractical and perhaps impossible. Too many vested financial or other interests will not readily relinquish their territory.

Still, in closing, I want to suggest here a rough blueprint for a way forward. Any short-term hopes for the medical system's fundamental reform—or even moderation—appear futile. I believe a better strategy involves ignoring the medical regime's official institutional structures whenever possible and building new ones—small-scale initiatives where decentralized medical care can be restored, and patients can be empowered to take responsibility for their own health. We need what the Czech dissidents of the 1970s called a "parallel polis" for medical institutions.[2] This would supplement the beneficial and necessary functions that are missing in the existing structures and, wherever possible, would use those existing structures and humanize them. These initiatives need not lead to a direct conflict with mainstream medical institutions—a conflict that the upstarts would, deprived of institutional power, certainly lose. At the same time, this strategy harbors no illusions that cosmetic changes to mainstream medicine can make much meaningful difference.

My proposed strategy involves first occupying the spaces that medicine has temporarily abandoned or which it never occupied in the first place. These parallel institutions need not constitute a ghetto or an underground; they are not a black-market system hiding in the shadows. The purpose of these institutions is to eventually renew the entire healthcare system, not to retreat from it entirely.[3]

Admittedly, every institution of the parallel polis will be a David facing the Goliath of a massively powerful and totalizing medical system. Any one or another of these institutions could be crushed by the state machinery, working as the enforcement arm of institutional and corporate medical power, if the state specifically targeted it for liquidation. Our task, therefore, is to create so many of these parallel structures and institutions that the captured state would finally be limited in its reach. While it could crush any one institution at any time, there would eventually be too many such initiatives for the state to target them all simultaneously.

At the behest of governments during the Covid crisis, medical institutions demanded we become disempowered and isolated, abandoning social solidarity. Governments weaponized fear to coerce individuals, families, and communities to cede their sovereignty and even make them forget they once had it. To help them reclaim their ability to self-govern, we must help people overcome their fear and find their courage.

The new parallel institutions of medicine must return sovereignty to individuals, families, and communities and strengthen social solidarity. These institutions should help people take responsibility for their health and must always support the doctor-patient relationship, minimizing external intrusions on this relationship. In these new medical models, physicians need to be able to exercise individualized clinical judgment and appropriate discretionary latitude. Doctors should work primarily for patients and only secondarily for institutions.

Markets, communications, and governing structures within medicine have become increasingly centralized at a national and global level, robbing individuals, families, and local communities of legitimate authority, privacy, and medical freedom. Thus, the new medical institutions must be grounded in technologies and models of decentralized communications and information-sharing, dispersed authority, and localized markets. To name just one example among many, subscription-based models of direct primary care, which bypass Medicare and other third-party payers, are springing up around the country, showing a twenty-fold increase in the last fifteen years.[4] In many cases these are proving financially viable—delivering better health outcomes at lower costs by axing the expensive and superfluous bureaucratic middlemen.[5] The Mercatus Center at George Mason University found in a 2021 analysis that direct primary care can reduce administrative financial overhead by approximately 40 percent, attributing this to the elimination of third-party insurance billing and associated compliance costs.[6]

Individuals, families, and local communities have been robbed of their legitimate authority. To rectify this, the new medical institutions must support the principle of subsidiarity and empower practical efforts at the local level. New member-owned cooperatives as an alternative to traditional health insurance are another example of recent creative thinking in the domain of healthcare reimbursements that respect this principle of subsidiarity, reduce administrative costs, and help individuals and families maintain legitimate authority over healthcare payments.[7] Other potentially promising examples could be multiplied, but my purpose here is not to enumerate all the initiatives that would go into making up a parallel polis for medicine, but merely to sketch the conceptual framework for such a movement.

Ultimately, we need to plant seeds that might not fully germinate in our lifetimes and think in fifty-year or one-hundred-year increments. Consider as a helpful analogy the homeschooling movement in the United States. In 1973, just over fifty years ago, there were thirteen thousand homeschoolers; today there are five million. A generation ago, parents would get a visit from social services for not sending their children to "approved" public or private schools. It was considered déclassé, if not borderline criminal, to attempt to educate one's children oneself.

Undeterred by suspicion and outright persecution, the homeschool movement created a parallel polis, reappropriating the idea of self-education and autonomous learning that had been monopolized by those with advanced degrees in education. While not every homeschooler succeeded, many thrived, demonstrating that their children could get a superior education—winning the spelling bees, acing standardized exams, and earning admission to prestigious universities—for a fraction of the cost of other schools. These pioneers formed co-ops, and often later founded private or charter schools, thereby influencing directly or indirectly the mainstream educational landscape. This movement eventually changed the face of institutional education. Homeschooling is now part of the mainstream, and the resources to facilitate it have multiplied.

Medicine today needs its own equivalent to the homeschool movement. Ordinary people need to reappropriate the idea of self-care and self-directed healing that has been monopolized by physicians and other healthcare professionals. Just as homeschooling deinstitutionalized education, so we need to demedicalize healthcare, at least to some extent. Medical professionals have our role, to be sure—just as professional teachers continue to have a role in influencing and often assisting the pioneers of homeschooling. But doctors and nurses need not be the only game in town. Over time, perhaps in fifty years, this decentralized healthcare movement will positively influence the practice of institutionalized medicine both directly and indirectly.

This kind of democratizing movement, empowering ordinary people to act independently in their own self-care, is not without historical precedent in American medicine. In the nineteenth century, practical books for the domestic practice of medicine enjoyed wide popularity.

According to Pulitzer Prize–winning historian of medicine Paul Starr, "Written in lucid, everyday language, avoiding Latin or technical terms, the books set forth current knowledge on disease and attacked, at times explicitly, the conception of medicine as a high mystery."[8] The most popular of these works was Dr. William Buchan's *Domestic Medicine*, which carried the tagline, "an attempt to render the Medical Art more generally useful, by showing people what is in their own power both with respect to the Prevention and Cure of Diseases." The book went through more than thirty editions in America between 1781 and the mid-1800s.

Although the author was a member of the Royal College of Physicians of Edinburgh, the most prestigious medical institution of the day, he was highly critical of the medical profession's monopolistic elitism, writing that "no discovery can ever be of general utility while the practice of it is kept in the hands of a few."[9] As Starr notes, "Though Buchan did not dismiss the value of physicians when they were available, he upheld the view that professional knowledge and training were unneeded in treating most diseases. . . . Most people, he assured readers, 'trust too little to their own endeavors.'"[10] Buchan maintained a general skepticism toward the value of drugs, preferring to focus on diet and preventive measures like the Hippocratic physicians of old. In his words, "I think the administration of medicines always doubtful, and often dangerous, and would much rather teach men how to avoid the necessity of using them, than how they should be used."[11] As Starr describes, "He counseled repeatedly that exercise, fresh air, a simple regimen, and cleanliness were of more value in maintaining health than anything medicine could do."[12] This remains as true today as when Buchan wrote in the nineteenth century.

Today, the specific medical content of these books is less instructive than the fact of their enormous popularity, which indicated a culture that generally embraced a model of autonomous self-care, with lay medical wisdom cultivated in the context of the family. This was likewise a period of intense iatrogenic medical injuries, when "mainstream" medicine's mainstays included harmful bloodletting and emetic purges for most diseases. Through these popularized works of domestic medicine, medical knowledge—such as it was at the time—and less aggressive medical interventions were democratized, decentralized, and made widely available to the broadest possible audience. Common sense was trusted to accomplish much of the necessary work, with physicians available when necessary for situations that the lay public could not manage.

In the realm of organized medicine, I'll mention just one example of a parallel, alternative medical society that I recently helped establish along with three other doctors from Duke, Harvard, and Stanford. The Hippocratic Society, which as of this writing has chapters for premedical and medical students at nine universities and counting, exists to form and sustain clinicians in the practice and pursuit of good medicine.[13] "HippSoc," as we nicknamed it, focuses on helping medical students and practicing physicians cultivate the virtues that characterize good medical practice. What passes for medical ethics today often asks doctors to set aside clinical judgment in service to the expectations of third parties or to patient "autonomy" arbitrarily defined. In contrast, Hippocratic Society physicians seek to discern and do what good medicine requires, thereby fulfilling our healing profession.

Today's corporatization of healthcare treats practitioners as interchangeable "providers" who are expected to "just do your job"—that is, do what the external managerial elites dictate—which contributes to a crisis of medical morale. The Hippocratic Society embraces medicine as a sacred profession in the service of the patient's genuine good. In our age of medical censorship, HippSoc also sponsors fair, serious, and open discourse about the most important questions facing medical practitioners in our time. Against the tendency in academia to ignore or suppress disagreement and dissent, this new medical society promotes public dialogue and debate about difficult questions in medicine. We are confident that by reasoning together, medical practitioners can discern better how to serve our patients and fulfill our profession.

If we succeed, every major academic medical center will have an active chapter of the Hippocratic Society by 2035. A dense network of senior clinicians will serve as mentors to medical trainees, and a parallel network of clinician chapters will support practitioners across the United States and beyond. The success of this enterprise will be measured not only by the number of chapters created or symposia held, but especially by the character and flourishing of the practitioners who participate in this community. We are confident that HippSoc members will be recognized by their peers and patients alike as exemplars of the medical profession—trustworthy healers characterized by knowledge and skill, wisdom and compassion, courage and integrity.

This is just one example among the hundreds of new medical institutions we need to begin building. If we fail to make the necessary reforms, young talent will be misdirected and their energies mismanaged. The loss will be incalculable. Iatrogenic harms from managerialized medicine will continue to multiply. This sobering and sometimes severe assessment of medicine's current crisis need not be the last word. There is hope. If we succeed in building parallel institutions that can help restore medicine, the gains will be worth every effort. Renewal is possible if we put our hand to the plow and do the work.

How can medical education contribute to the necessary reforms? Many people today complain that their physician cannot relate to them, does not have time for them, or fails to address their real concerns. Their doctor sometimes seems more like a technician or an impersonal manager than a companion or confidant. He or she may have plenty of know-how, but something else is missing. What patients desire in a doctor is a person not only of knowledge and skill, but also someone they can relate to, a person of character and goodwill. Are medical schools today failing to inculcate the necessary virtues in their students? Is it possible for them to do so? Socrates raised a similar question over two thousand years ago: Can virtue be taught? If so, how?

Medical school puts a premium on the virtues of knowledge, prudence, perseverance, industriousness, efficiency, and so on, while neglecting other necessary virtues. Some have suggested that med schools should add courses in the arts and humanities so that doctors "can relate to their patients" better. As you probably gathered from my writing, I appreciate the arts and humanities as much as anyone—indeed, I was among the three faculty founders of the Center for Medical Humanities at UCI—but I suspect this is only part of the answer. Piling Shakespeare and Vincent van Gogh on top of an already overloaded medical curriculum is a tough sell, and study of the humanities alone will not automatically make someone more humanistic or compassionate.

Medical students must bring wisdom and humanistic qualities to the table when they arrive at medical school. Students must take an active interest in all things human, without needing to be force-fed these subjects. It is too late, once in medical school, to inculcate all the qualities of a good physician in someone whose outlook and interests are narrow at the outset. The difficult task of selection and admission of students includes finding those whose talents and interests go beyond scientific pursuits, as important as those clearly are for medicine. Pre-med requirements were recently broadened to include more social sciences. Expanding them to the humanities could be another salutary development, though the humanities remain impoverished by ideology or general neglect at most undergraduate institutions.[14]

Although increasingly deployed today, a doomed approach involves attempts to ensure medical students' professional competence through more testing, additional accreditation requirements, and more bureaucratic watchdogs. Although utilized more frequently than medical humanities classes, this managerialist approach to medical education is futile. Writing mission statements, vision statements, competency requirements; developing tracking systems, patient logs, disciplinary policies; and conducting seminars in customer satisfaction, interpersonal skills, and communication methods—all this generally amounts to so many reams of paper and so much empty talk. Rules and regulations, techniques and strategies—these may occasionally help prevent the worst from happening, but they do not bring out the best in people. What medical schools need first are motivated students of ability and generosity. And, of course, they need talented teachers.

Every medical student knows a few teaching physicians that he seeks to imitate—doctors who were instrumental in shaping the course of his medical education. Every doctor that I worked under, both the admirable and the less than admirable, shaped who I am today. Sometimes I learned what I wanted to avoid doing as a doctor, but far more often I noticed some trait, some habit, some virtue that I hoped to emulate. "Doctor" literally means "teacher": The finest physicians were also the best educators. I formed my notion of the ideal physician from a composite of actual physicians that I learned from and admired during my training. I came to appreciate that the ideal physician combines apparently contradictory qualities—he possesses virtues that remain in tension with one another.

The same doctor who is stirred to his depths by a patient in distress must also possess the calm detachment to diagnose the source of distress and quickly administer the appropriate remedy. He must simultaneously be the warm companion and the cool observer; he must be attached in heart and detached in mind; he must learn to remain calm amidst chaos. "This calm gives the doctor the eye that will penetrate, undimmed by tears; it lets the surgeon operate with hands that do not tremble," wrote Karl Jaspers. "It is a great challenge to keep a warm heart in this coolness."[15] Intimacy and distance: Effective doctors hold both these polarities in a balanced and fruitful tension.

Similarly, the physician should be both a scientist and more than a scientist. He must possess knowledge of, and unflagging confidence in, the discoveries of his science. At the same time, he must remain fully aware of the limits of modern science and the dangers of putting all his faith and hope in scientific progress. Biological and psychological sciences have undoubtedly taught me much about human beings, for which I am grateful. But for all their successes and triumphs, the natural sciences are silent with respect to the ultimate concerns raised by my patients and by my experiences in medical school.

I say this not just to raise the standard humanist objection that science is too impersonal, detached, or logical—that it ignores human art, culture, or faith, and so forth. Rather, modern science fails when it claims to be all-encompassing, when it promises to give a complete picture of man and the universe. The novelist Walker Percy was fond of pointing this out, as a physician and admirer of science, not merely as a critic; in his words, he was setting himself up not as the small boy noticing the naked emperor, but as someone whispering to a friend at a party that he would do well to fix his fly.[16] Percy argued that modern science accounts for pretty well everything in the universe except for man—his peculiar self, which always remains a "leftover" in any comprehensive scientific system.

In short: Science explains everything except what it means to be a particular person in this world, to be born, and to die. But particular people—with all their foibles and follies, and with all their transcendent aspirations and achievements—are precisely the recipients and the providers of medical care. Science is clearly an essential component of the practice of medicine, but it is only one component, for it cannot answer the ultimate questions that confront us most forcefully when we experience the extremes of life—extremes such as illness, bodily affliction, and death. Science is a great boon, and it constitutes the foundation for medicine; but scientism—the (nonscientific) claim that science is the only valid form of knowledge—is a false idol that corrupts medicine.

Medical school could be significantly improved by more direct observation of students' interactions with patients. We students were typically evaluated on what we told the other doctors after we had seen the patient. I can remember only a few occasions where a resident or attending actually watched me interact, through an interview or just an ordinary conversation, with a patient. I could have been a blockhead at the bedside, and this would not have affected my medical school grades in the least.

Our grades rarely included an assessment of this intangible something that patients call "bedside manner." Evaluations were based instead upon our ability to answer pimp questions, our willingness to do scut work, and our readiness to stay after-hours (if there was indeed such a thing as "work hours"). Above all, we were evaluated on the rapidity with which we carried out tasks. When the workload was heavy, busy residents placed a premium on efficiency. There is nothing inherently wrong with working efficiently; it is often very necessary. But in the end, patients care little about how efficient their doctor is. I suspect most patients prefer a doctor or medical student who inefficiently "wasted" more of his precious time talking with them.

For a medical student, praise from superiors was faint, blame frequent. Like the center on the football team, almost no one notices when you do your job well, but everyone sees when you fumble the snap. More than once, I was caught in the trap of trying to look good mostly to please my superiors. I gradually came to realize that this was fruitless. Such eager-to-please students wait like a dog, panting for their master to throw a few scraps of encouragement from his table above. The highest praise I could hope to receive from a resident was the coveted phrase, "strong work."

Initially, this was sweet music to my ears. *What joy!* "Strong work," I would repeat to myself, bustling down the hall with a new spring in my tired step. But like a drug, the effect of this praise soon wore off, and I would have to go in search of my next hit. The med student who becomes addicted to compliments from colleagues soon finds himself desperately craving a substance that is found only in short supply. This cannot be the pathway toward career satisfaction, I eventually decided. What, then, was the real source of professional satisfaction in medical school? In other words, why did I choose this career and why did I stay in it?

During the times of serious doubt, when I would systematically tally up the pros and cons, I would nearly become convinced that I should have opted for another profession. On the face of it, choosing medical school seemed ludicrous. It was long, expensive, and exhausting. The hospital hierarchy was dizzying and confusing, with myself as the student fixed firmly at the bottom. I was often scutted, pimped, and even exploited for my eagerness to please. I was sleep-deprived, food-deprived, and leisure-deprived. Prudence dictated that I should have cut my losses and walked away. I am glad that I did not.

My doubts were often influenced not by dislike for the practice of medicine, but by physical exhaustion, by fear of making a mistake when patients' lives were at stake, by frustration with the current healthcare system, and by the stress and strain of medical training. When I was tempted to abandon medical school, I would try to step back from my troubles to gain a more objective view. I realized that in my weighing of the pros and cons, I had taken for granted many things that could be summarized by this obvious fact: Being a physician is an enormous privilege.

Society places high expectations upon doctors in exchange for the extraordinary opportunities granted us. Given this commission to heal, I had a serious responsibility to live up to the standards to which physicians are held. I was being groomed for tasks of enormous consequence for the lives of others. Because of what physicians are expected to do to and for people, training for this should not have been easy, should not have been without pain and struggle. Although my complaints were sometimes legitimate, they needed to be weighed on the balance against the duty and dispensation that come with being a doctor.

I had been given the opportunity to become a physician. When I finally grasped that this was an undertaking of considerable gravity and magnitude, I found the stamina to continue. To be a doctor—to be granted invasive access to a person's body and mind, to be responsible for administering the potentially hazardous healing arts without doing harm—was a privilege that rightly called for years of *hard* training. I needed to rise to the occasion if I wanted to don the doctor's mantle. Looking back, the memories of the hardships fade. What remains is the satisfaction, the exhilaration of having run the race and finished.

If I had walked away, I never would have known the thrill of pulling a bleeding patient back from the brink. I never would have placed a newborn son into the hands of his mother for the first time. I never would have known the joy of telling a terminally ill patient that today she will receive a new organ that will save her life, never have felt this patient grasp my hand, or seen the radiance in her face as tears welled up. I never would have tasted the sorrow of touching a dying patient with an act of mercy that restored him, if only for a moment, to his vocation. Finally, had I chosen another path, I never would have felt the deep chord struck within me by the patients who simply said, "Thank you, Doctor." These words, and not words of praise from my superiors, were the true source of fulfillment in medical school.

Why do we do it? The answer is simple: We do it for the patients. Those of us who are called to this profession are drawn ultimately by the opportunity to help heal another human being. There were a few remarkable and extraordinary patients who made everything worthwhile, who repaid my efforts a hundredfold. They were the reason that medical school was the toughest job that I could not live without. They were the reasons I chose to persevere and why I am grateful I made the cut.

CONCLUSION

To the Wonder

We shall not cease from exploration
And the end of all our exploring
Will be to arrive where we started
And know the place for the first time.
            —T. S. Eliot, "Little Gidding"[1]

I was only just beginning when I walked the graduation stage over twenty years ago and received the *Medicinae Doctoris* degree (Georgetown diplomas still used the Latin). Things did not actually get easier as a resident, or later as an attending physician, but they did get better. The stakes became progressively higher, the stress often more intense. But the rewards became more personal, the patients more my own. My work has brought me into close contact with a cross-section of humanity rarely encountered in most occupations. My patients have ranged from physicians and priests to prostitutes and porn performers, from homeless derelicts and ex-convicts to billionaire trust-funders and brilliant scholars—each of them in their own way fascinating and frustrating, inspiring and beguiling.

After graduation, I completed four years of residency training in psychiatry at the University of California, Irvine. When I finished, I stayed on to join the faculty there, where I served for sixteen years as professor in the School of Medicine and as director of the medical ethics program in the hospital. I taught courses across all four years of the medical school curriculum and spent several years as residency training director and clerkship director in psychiatry. In my work in medical education, I found myself gradually moving back to the beginning, devoting more time to teaching medical students earlier in their training.

I confess, I enjoyed the first-year students the most—the ones who approach this whole enterprise with fresh eyes. I saw my own experiences reflected in theirs, and I saw in their stories the kind of stories I've told here. These first-years kept me close to my first loves as a physician: learning something entirely new about the body or the brain and seeing a new patient for the first time. There is always the danger for physicians that our initial wonder turns to cynicism, that our early enthusiasm gives way to burnout. The first-year medical students—excited, terrified, grateful, overwhelmed, hopeful, timid—remind me that I too am still a beginner. And they remind me why I was drawn to this profession in the first place.

I vividly recall the day when it really sunk in that I was no longer the medical student, no longer the intern or resident, but was finally the attending physician. It suddenly struck me that, as the attending, I was the one ultimately responsible for the welfare of the patients in my charge, the final locus of responsibility through which help or harm came to the patient.

It was my first week as the new attending psychiatrist directing an eighteen-bed locked acute inpatient psychiatric unit. One of the patients was a towering, hefty man who suffered from chronic schizophrenia and severe paranoid thinking. James had become increasingly agitated during this hospitalization. That day, when his lab results were (in his estimation) late in returning, his agitation reached a fevered pitch. He stormed over to the locked door of the ward and, with a yell, began kicking the door with all his might. The door rattled under the force of his boot as he repeatedly reared back and laid into it with all his 260 pounds of heft.

The nurses picked up the phone to call security for help. The rest of us froze for a second or two, staring dumbfounded as he laid into the door, which creaked and groaned on its hinges with blow after blow. Somewhere around the ninth or tenth kick, the door gave way and burst open. *Wait a minute . . . this was supposed to be a "locked unit,"* I thought. I had never imagined that someone could kick the door down.

On the other side of the psychiatric unit door was the ARU—the Acute Rehabilitation Unit—a non-psychiatric ward where frail patients in walkers hobbled slowly while they recovered from strokes and other injuries. James sauntered through the busted-open door into the ARU. I knew that security would still be minutes away from arriving. Instantly, I realized there was no one else on the unit to look to for help; I was now the attending physician. It was up to me to do something. Acting purely on instinct, and without a well-formulated plan, I ran across the unit and through the open door. Looking to my left, I saw James. Probably too stunned by his success to know what to do once he escaped, he had stopped momentarily at a water fountain to take a drink.

"James," I said, placing my hand gently on his elbow. "You need to come with me back to 1 North." He paused and stared blankly down at me for a moment, not saying a word. The rage appeared to have subsided from his eyes, replaced by a look of befuddled confusion. "You need to come with me," I repeated, and began walking slowly, leading him by the elbow back through the door. He had probably been as surprised as the rest of us when the door flew open, and didn't really have a plan for what came next after leaving the unit. To my grateful astonishment, he put up no resistance and walked with me in silence back to 1 North. It took me an hour or two before the adrenaline cleared from my system and the tremors in my hands subsided.

After this incident, the hospital installed steel-reinforced double doors to reduce the AWOL risk. Despite our best safety measures, there is no contingency plan for everything that happens in medicine. Sometimes the last thing you expect just happens, and in those moments the physicians need to act, or react, using our best instincts. I have no idea what I would have done had James refused to accompany me back or if he had commenced rampaging around the ARU. What I did know in that split second after he disappeared through the busted-open doorway was this: I needed to do something. There was no one else to look to; the buck stopped with me. In the hospital hierarchy, I had moved from the bottom of the totem pole to the top. Of course, I was now perched in the place I had for so many years aspired to reach, but now that I had arrived, I realized that things are sometimes lonely there. At the top, there are fewer people to look to for guidance or to share the burdens of the work.

Practicing medicine has changed me, as it changes all physicians. Our work profoundly shapes our perceptions of people and of the world in ways we probably don't even realize. The contemporary philosopher Thomas Nagel wrote a widely cited and influential paper about subjective mental experiences titled "What Is It Like to Be a Bat?"[2] For me, trying to imagine what it would have been like *not* to go through medical school and *not* to practice medicine is sort of like trying to imagine what it is like to be a bat. Just as fatherhood is central to who I am, medicine is now a foundational part of my identity. Having a child forever changes you; there is simply no going back, as any parent knows. Medical school and the practice of medicine have likewise changed me irreversibly. As my story suggests, it was often a painful ordeal. But the pain fades. We forget, like a new mother who quickly forgets the pain of labor with the joy of giving birth.

Medicine has changed me mostly for this reason: My patients are now an intrinsic part of who I am. Their lives are inextricably intertwined with mine. My own happiness and success are no longer a separate project, somehow standing apart from my patients' well-being. I have been placed in the often charged, always challenging, frequently sad center of my patients' lives. In the process, my patients have taught me more than anyone else about medicine, about suffering, about resilience, and about hope. More than any textbook, more than my professors in medical school, and more than my mentors in residency, my patients have been my best teachers.

In the end, mine is not a tale of cynicism or mere critique, but of wonder. Medicine, for all its limitations and problems and hardships, is still a wondrous enterprise. The stories we physicians become a part of are usually messy—because life itself is messy—and the outcomes are often mixed. Occasionally, there are extremely painful moments when our patients or their families look at us with contempt and even derision, where we feel that we have failed them. But far more often than not, the patients and families look at us with gratitude. And that is enough.

Early in my tenure as an attending physician, I saw a patient of mine in the clinic, a young woman who had been under my care for several years. Over the past weeks, her mental state had taken a turn for the worse, and she was for the first time acutely manic and becoming increasingly agitated. At one point during our session, she impulsively stood up, grabbed my notes out of my hand, and tore them up. After trying to reason with her to no avail, I decided that she needed to be hospitalized in order to stabilize her manic symptoms, since she appeared to be a potential danger to others. Needless to say, the patient was not pleased with this, and security had to be called in to assist.

I went to the waiting room to speak with her worried father, who had driven her to the clinic that day. "I have never seen her like this," he said. "I don't know what's going on. She is not acting like herself."

I explained my decision to hospitalize her and my recommendation to initiate a mood stabilizing medication. I tried to reassure him that her condition would improve with treatment.

"Are you sure we need to hospitalize her?" he asked me. "She has never been hospitalized before, and she will not be happy about this. Are you sure it's the right decision?"

"Yes, I am sure," I replied. "I have dealt with many cases like hers. This is what she needs now. It's the best thing for her." My confidence in this decision was growing by the moment, though nothing in medicine is certain. Physicians learn to live with a seed of doubt in the back of our minds that serves to remind us that our clinical judgments are not infallible. With the patient's father, however, I proceeded with the steady calm and confidence that physicians are expected to maintain when managing a crisis. "We will take good care of her," I reassured him. "I believe that she'll be looking more like herself within a few days of treatment."

He looked directly at me. "I don't know what to do," he said. "But I trust you . . ."

To become worthy of this trust, and to remain faithful to this trust, is the aspiration of every student who enters medical school and dons the physician's white coat.

With admiration and gratitude for all modern medicine's technological wizardry, I believe that at the heart of medicine we still find (and always will find) not a new technology or a novel technique, but a relationship—indeed, a relationship of a very distinctive kind, as we explored in chapter 8 in the discussion of the doctor-patient relationship. None of the great apparatus of modern medicine—the hospitals with their complex buzz of activity, the MRI scanners that can visualize small anomalies in the body, the precision surgical robots, the wonder drugs, the intricate machinery of medical education, the vast sums of money spent on the whole enterprise—none of this exists for the medical students or the physicians. Neither is it for the hospital administrators, nor the insurance company executives, nor the politicians trying to devise workable healthcare policies.

At the end of the day, medicine is only about that person lying there in the hospital bed, or nervously walking into the clinic, or anxiously awaiting her test results. The entire enterprise has always been about, and will always be about, the patients. Physician competence is a necessary but never sufficient condition for good medical care. As Sir Francis Peabody put it in a famous address to the students at Harvard Medical School in 1926: The secret to the care of the patient is in *caring* for the patient.[3]

Occasionally, when I could free up an hour or two in the afternoon, I invited the third-year medical students on the psychiatry clerkship to participate in a "jam session" for the patients on the acute inpatient psychiatric unit. We typically scraped together just enough musical talent to manage well enough, and a few portable instruments to play—usually an acoustic guitar or two, perhaps a keyboard or some tambourines. Then we did our best to provide a little levity and distraction for the hospitalized patients. Some faculty may think this is a corny "Patch Adams" ruse, an unserious waste of time for a medical educator. But the students—and more importantly, the patients—typically loved it. It allowed the students to see the patients in a different mode, and it allowed the patients to relate to students and faculty in a context that was more relaxed.

One jam session featured me on the guitar and vocals (just barely holding down the tune and lamely strumming a few chords), a more talented student on keyboard, another on electric guitar, and a few shy students providing backup vocals. We commenced with one of the few songs I had in my limited repertoire, and as we began to play, the patients made their way out of their rooms and over to the common area to hear this curiosity. When I hit the chorus of Leonard Cohen's "Hallelujah," a nineteen-year-old patient named Maria suddenly began belting out the lyrics in a perfect harmony: "*It's a cold and it's a broken Hallelujah . . .*"[4]

Her voice was stunning. Nurses began congregating to hear where this singing was coming from, and everyone broke out in spontaneous applause when Maria finished the song. We followed with the Imagine Dragons song "Demons" (covering both ends of the spiritual spectrum, I suppose), which Maria also sang with aplomb.

As the second round of applause died away, another patient shuffled over, leaned in, and quietly asked me, "Can I play your guitar?" He was a bearded young man, disheveled and dressed in a hospital gown and socks. I figured this fellow just wanted to share some of the limelight that Maria was enjoying.

"What's your name?" I inquired.

"Joe. I'm homeless." He looked the part. "I play on the streets."

"Sure, no problem, Joe," I said, handing him the guitar. I wasn't yet sure what he was going to do with it or if I would get it back in one piece. But within seconds, it was clear that Joe played the guitar even better than Maria sang. The rest of the hour was their show. Maria would suggest a song she liked, and Joe somehow knew how to play every tune—the Beatles, Zeppelin, Metallica, Tom Petty, Incubus, Oasis, Green Day. The usually dull psychiatric ward came alive. The students and I sat back with the patients and nurses and took it in. Joe eventually moved from the acoustic to the electric guitar, where his talents were even more apparent as his fingers moved up and down the neck of the guitar in a blazing, finger-tapping solo that would have made Jimi Hendrix proud.

Between songs, I asked Joe if he was in a band.

"Used to be," he said. "Not anymore. Drugs."

"If you can get clean," I told him, "you can do just about anything you want musically."

"I know," he smiled. "Getting clean is the hard part."

Joe was reluctant to relinquish the guitar when it was time for us to wrap up. Maria clasped my hand and thanked me with tears for bringing the instruments into the unit. Joe and Maria had ended their jam session that day with "Home" by Phillip Phillips of *American Idol* fame. If circumstances had been different, it was not hard to imagine these two patients up on that stage under the bright lights, with Joe strumming and Maria singing, "*Just know you're not alone, cause I'm gonna make this place your home . . .*"[5]

The medical students were beaming as we walked off the unit that day. When you're the doctor, it's easy to forget, or fail to notice, that your patients are extraordinary people.

A few years ago, I evaluated a seventy-nine-year-old man referred to me by a colleague. Mr. Chong had immigrated from China many years ago, and by dint of hard work he had achieved professional success and provided well for his wife and three children, who were now grown and themselves professionally successful. This patient had initially presented to our medical school's willed body program, with the intent to donate his body to science immediately after his death. Things proceeded normally with this process until he told the person taking down his information the *precise date*—approximately one year in the future—when his body would be donated to the University. Puzzled, the employee inquired further, only to learn that Mr. Chong had an unusual plan in mind.

He intended to come to our hospital on a predetermined day, where he would (so he hoped) receive a lethal injection of a medication from a physician. His healthy and fresh organs and tissues could then be immediately harvested and donated to research, or perhaps used for transplantation. All neat, clean, and tidy. Nonplussed with his plan, the dean's office referred him to our psychiatric department for consultation. He had come to the appointment hoping to find a physician who would administer to him a lethal drug on this predetermined date. "Doctor," he pleaded with me during our initial visit, "please help me to do this."

The first psychiatrist to see him could find no signs or symptoms of a mental disorder, and so recommended that he see a psychiatric resident who shared Mr. Chong's ethnic background, to try to determine if there were perhaps cultural factors influencing his unusual decision. The resident could likewise find nothing wrong in terms of a psychiatric disorder but could also make little sense of his plan for suicide; he also denied any culture-specific factors influencing this plan. So together they referred him to me—the medical ethicist and psychiatrist—mostly out of desperation and befuddlement. "See what you can make of this," they told me. "We can't find anything wrong with him, but he is very set on this suicide plan."

In our first session, Mr. Chong explained to me that he believed—though he did not have definitive proof—that his father and grandfather had both died by suicide on their sixtieth birthdays, and he seemed to suggest there was some precedent for this practice in Chinese culture. His internet-based research had somehow led him to the conclusion that he could find a physician in the United States to help him do this. "Euthanasia," he explained, "I've read about it." With each subsequent consultation with physicians in our department, Mr. Chong continued to nurture the hope that some doctor from our institution would assist him in dying by suicide before he turned eighty. Part of my role was to disabuse him of this notion. But first, I wanted to drill down deeper and try to figure out exactly why he was so determined to end his life.

If he was still in good health, why would he turn in his ticket at eighty? The fixed date seemed arbitrary. This intelligent and successful man explained to me that he had accomplished all he wanted to do in life, that he wished to leave this world before he developed any serious medical problems and before he had to possibly endure a slow decline or period of disability, and that he did not want to risk someday becoming a burden on his family. "I don't want to bother anyone," he said repeatedly.

The idea of death by suicide did not appear to frighten him in the least; but I could find no symptoms of depression, anxiety, psychosis, or other mental health problems. He was in remarkably robust physical health for his age, which he acknowledged. Knowing in advance the reason for the referral, to my surprise he impressed me as a warm, good-natured, cheerful man. I found it easy to like him almost immediately. With his characteristic optimism, he seemed rather dismissive of my suggestion that his self-inflicted death could have a lasting negative emotional impact on his wife and three adult children. The potential impact on his family was the one piece that did not seem to fit, the part where the story did not quite add up. So I recommended a follow-up session with his family members to get their perspective, and the patient agreed to this.

Mr. Chong arrived at the follow-up visit impeccably dressed but wore sunglasses throughout the entire session. I believe these served the purpose of masking his emotions in the presence of his son, who accompanied him. As it turned out, his wife, daughter, and one of his sons refused to attend. The other son who did accompany him clearly expressed frustration and anger towards his father. "I told him I am opposed to his suicide plan, but I'm tired of arguing with him about it," the son explained. He also informed me that for many years Mr. Chong's relationship with his wife and children had been strained. One of his sons refused to speak with him, and his wife slept in a separate bedroom. As we unpacked the family dynamics during this session, the patient eventually admitted to having long-standing issues with anger, which had adversely affected his familial relationships. Mr. Chong explained that he felt misunderstood by his family, and that he had lost control over them and lost the respect of his children.

When he continued to persist in his suicide plan, I explained that physician-assisted suicide was illegal in California (it still was at that time) and, furthermore, that my colleagues and I considered it to be unethical. I explained that no willed body program in the United States would accept the donation of a body from someone who had taken his own life, as these institutions would not want to encourage suicidal acts. Gradually, the reality sunk in that he would not be able to donate his body to science if he ended his own life. He appeared deflated. No medical school would help him purchase redemption for his untimely death by accepting his donated cadaver.

On the other hand, it was helpful for him to hear me explain that he still had the right to refuse medical care in the future—that the informed refusal of medical interventions was not equivalent to a deliberate attempt to take his own life. "Refusing excessively burdensome medical care simply means allowing a disease to take its natural course," I told him. "This is medically and morally different from doing something to deliberately kill oneself."

His son nodded his head vigorously. "That's what I've been trying to tell him."

Mr. Chong seemed comforted when I assured him that physicians would respect his wishes if he decided in the future to refuse burdensome or useless medical interventions. He appeared relieved with the thought that he could still exercise that degree of autonomy at the end of his life. While his medical future—as is true for all of us—was to some extent uncertain, he would not necessarily be consigned to die an unduly prolonged or undignified death.

In my interpretation, suicide was an escape hatch for this patient, an easy way out of having to do the hard work of attempting to repair and reconcile broken familial relationships. It was an ultimate and definitive means of avoidance. His son explained that he believed suicide was a selfish act, and he agreed that his father's self-inflicted death would indeed have a longstanding adverse impact on the family. Together we explained to Mr. Chong that ending his life would prematurely and definitively foreclose the possibility of ever trying to reconcile and improve these relationships. Those who survived him would have to live the remainder of their days with these regrets. At some point during these discussions, a light—at least a dim light—appeared to go on. We began to see some chinks in his armor. Something we said struck a chord with him.

As the session concluded, Mr. Chong started to indicate that, if our hospital and our physicians would not help him euthanize himself, perhaps he would consider abandoning his plan to end his life. By the conclusion of the session with his son, he even indicated a furtive willingness to attempt the hard and humbling work of amending and reconciling the relationships with his estranged family members. I told him that I would make myself available for ongoing psychotherapy sessions to help him with this, if he was interested. "Maybe someday I'll call you," he said with a subtle smile.

I do not know what happened to Mr. Chong in the end. I never saw him again. I wonder, did I really discern a subtle turn in the direction of his life—the seeds of a willingness to press on in the face of a risky, unknown, and uncertain future? Naturally, I would like to hope that my interventions played a role in saving this man's life, helping both him and his family. But of course, I could be mistaken and just comforting myself with wishful thinking. The final outcome of this case—indeed, the outcome of most the cases I treat—is uncertain.

This kind of uncertainty is a permanent feature of medical practice. Society often views the physician as an authority figure, as someone who can confidently and consistently administer the right solutions for serious problems. But through hard experiences, the honest physician knows that this is typically an idealized fantasy. An experienced doctor must learn to live with uncertainty and inevitable limitations. The only way to proceed in the work of healing is to press forward, all the while recognizing that we might fail, that we might inadvertently make the wrong judgment call, and that the patient might not respond as we predict.

We are sustained by hope, not by certainties, because in medicine, there simply are no guarantees. Practicing medicine is therefore a kind of act of faith, and every physician struggles with doubts. What if I'm not up to the task? What if, despite my best efforts, the patient does not respond or recover? What if I make a costly mistake that harms my patient? What if another physician could have succeeded where I failed? What if the hopes this patient has placed in me are ultimately unfounded?

In countless interviews while serving on medical school or residency admissions committees over the years, I have asked applicants, "Why do you want to be a physician?" The typical answer is almost invariably something along the lines of, "Because I want to help people." That's all for the good, and, of course, it's indispensable in this line of work. But it's also not enough. If you want to be a doctor, then naturally you want to help people. But are you also ready to live with inescapable limits—with the failure to help people in some cases, or with the inability to help them in other cases? Are you prepared to endure the rather helpless experience of watching someone you have cared for grow worse or even die, despite your best efforts to help and to heal? Patients may often believe, or may nurture the hope, that the physician has all the answers they seek. But the seasoned physician, humbled by experience, knows otherwise.

If a bright and eager undergraduate student were to ask me, "How do I know if I am called to be a physician?" there are some suggestions and some questions I would pose for her consideration. To be a physician means to accompany patients through the enigmas of human life, death, suffering, and healing without having the power to resolve these enigmas. Indeed, the power of the physician today is paradoxically both immense and miniscule. This power is frequently astonishing in its ability to heal temporarily; but it is ultimately powerless in the face of death, which always has the last word in every medical case history.

Do you want to be a physician, to be among those who step into this breach? Then consider whether you can live and work every day within these tensions or between these polarities—and yet still maintain your warmth, equanimity, and hope. Consider whether you can live and work every day amid these paradoxes and challenges—and yet still cultivate the professional skill, the human kindness and compassion, that suffering patients always seek in the person that they call their doctor.

Acknowledgments

I did not complete medical school alone. My wife, Jennifer, as you can probably surmise from our year of medical mishaps described in chapter 8 and my own wavering as a medical student, was then and is now a most extraordinary person. When I doubted my abilities, she believed that I could finish, though she never forced me to stay in the race. While in medical school, marriage was my saving grace; without Jennifer, I would not have become a physician. Because its demands are often all-consuming, it is easy for students to get wrapped up entirely in the rigors of medical school. After a twelve-hour day of studying, it is common to go home to other medical student roommates and talk only about medicine. After thirty-six straight hours at the hospital, it is common to go home to the comfort of a bed and forget about the world outside. Family life kept me from being completely consumed by medical school. Jennifer was my anchor; she endured as many difficulties as I did during those long four years. For this, and for much else, I thank her.

My parents, Larry and Elaine, gave me everything a kid could hope for and more. As a psychiatrist who sees many patients who were deprived of a happy and secure childhood, I now appreciate this tremendous treasure they provided me—something I simply took for granted growing up. They remain my biggest cheerleaders, and I hope I have made them proud.

I want to thank my intrepid agent Jonathan Bronitsky at Athos, who championed this manuscript, and my thoughtful editor Kathryn Riggs at Regnery who believed in the manuscript and helped bring it into its final form. Without them, this book would not have finally seen the light of day over twenty years after I began working on it. A heartfelt thank you as well to Ryan Anderson, Mitch Muncy, and all my talented and generous colleagues at the Ethics and Public Policy Center, which has been the ideal home for my research and policy work after leaving academic medicine. Thank you also to my friend Jeffrey Tucker, founding director of the Brownstone Institute, for his unfailing support and for spurring me to resurrect this manuscript and pursue publication.

I am grateful to the attendings, fellows, and residents who taught me during medical school and residency. Medicine still operates mostly on an apprenticeship model of clinical training, and I was blessed with many exceptionally good mentors. I am likewise grateful for my colleagues during my years at the university as an attending physician, the excellent doctors who continued to teach me about the practice of medicine. I am grateful for the students and residents there that I had the privilege to teach, and from whom I learned a great deal more than they might suspect.

Finally, I am grateful to my patients. Whatever the problems that currently beset our healthcare system, my patients continue to give me courage and reasons for hope. They are the reason I still practice medicine with immense gratitude for the privilege of caring for them.

Notes

INTRODUCTION

1. Gerard Manley Hopkins, *Poems of Gerard Manley Hopkins*, ed. Robert Bridges (London: Humphrey Milford, 1918).
2. *Missouri v. Biden*, no. 3:22-cv-01213, 2023 WL 4335270 (W.D. La. July 4, 2023).
3. G. K. Chesterton, *What's Wrong with the World* (San Francisco: Ignatius Press, 1994), 190.
4. Karl Jaspers, *Philosophy and the World: Selected Essays and Lectures* (Washington: Regnery Gateway, 1989), 164.
5. Cormac McCarthy, *No Country for Old Men* (New York: Knopf, 2005), 63.
6. Jaspers, *Philosophy and the World*, 164.
7. Cited in Paul W. Brand and Philip Yancey, *Fearfully and Wonderfully Made: A Surgeon Looks at the Human and Spiritual Body* (Grand Rapids: Zondervan, 1980), 68. The first author attended the lecture where Mead provided this answer.
8. R. H. Perlis, K. Ognyanova, A. Uslu, et al., "Trust in Physicians and Hospitals During the COVID-19 Pandemic in a 50-State Survey of US Adults," *JAMA* Network Open 7, no. 7 (July 2024): e2424984, https://doi.org/10.1001/jamanetworkopen.2024.24984.
9. Brian Kennedy, Alec Tyson, and Cary Funk, "Americans' Trust in Scientists, Other Groups Declines," Pew Research Center, February 15, 2022, https://www.pewresearch.org/science/2022/02/15/americans-trust-in-scientists-other-groups-declines/.
10. US Centers for Disease Control and Prevention, "About Chronic Diseases," CDC.gov, October 4, 2024, https://www.cdc.gov/chronic-disease/about/index.html. Compare with Christine Buttorff, Teague Ruder, and Melissa Bauman, "Multiple Chronic Conditions in the United States," RAND Corporation, May 26, 2017, https://www.rand.org/pubs/tools/TL221.html.
11. Kathleen M. Harris, Malay K. Majmundar, and Tara Becker, eds., *High and Rising Mortality Rates among Working-Age Adults* (Washington: The National Academies Press, 2021), https://doi.org/10.17226/25976. "Already ranked relatively low in life expectancy (26th) in 2015 among the 35 countries that make up the Organisation for Economic Co-operation and Development, the United States would lose even more ground in its global position in national health and well-being."
12. Tanya Albert Henry, "Medicine's Great Resignation? 1 in 5 Doctors Plan Exit in 2 Years," American Medical Association, January 18,

2022, https://www.ama-assn.org/practice-management/physician-health/medicine-s-great-resignation-1-5-doctors-plan-exit-2-years.
13 K. J. Gold, A. Sen, and T. L. Schwenk, "Details on Suicide Among US Physicians: Data from the National Violent Death Reporting System," *General Hospital Psychiatry* 35, no. 1 (2013): 45–49, https://doi.org/10.1016/j.genhosppsych.2012.08.005.

CHAPTER 1

1 Sting, "Fragile," . . . *Nothing Like the Sun*, A&M Records, 1987.
2 E. Richard Brown, *Rockefeller Medicine Men: Medicine and Capitalism in America* (Berkeley: University of California Press, 1979), 119.
3 Catherine D. DeAngelis, "Big Pharma Profits and the Public Loses," *The Milbank Quarterly* 94, no. 11 (2016): 30–33, https://doi.org/10.1111/1468-0009; Sulagna Misra, "Medicine for Profit: The Pharmaceutical Industry's Stronghold and Impact on Patient Wellness," Medical Economics, October 14, 2024, https://www.medicaleconomics.com/view/medicine-for-profit-the-pharmaceutical-industry-s-stronghold-and-impact-on-patient-wellness; Fran Quigley, "Profits over Patients," *Prescription for the People: An Activist's Guide to Making Medicine Affordable for All* (Ithaca: Cornell University Press, 2017), 35–68, https://doi.org/10.7591/cornell/9781501713750.003.0007.
4 Tae Kim, "Goldman Sachs Asks in Biotech Research Report: 'Is Curing Patients a Sustainable Business Model?'," CNBC, April 11, 2018, https://www.cnbc.com/2018/04/11/goldman-asks-is-curing-patients-a-sustainable-business-model.html.

CHAPTER 2

1 Coldplay, "The Scientist," *A Rush of Blood to the Head*, Parlophone Records, 2022.
2 His real name.
3 E. D. Pellegrino, "Toward a Reconstruction of Medical Morality," *The Journal of Medical Humanities and Bioethics* 8 (March 1987): 7–18, https://doi.org/10.1007/BF01119343.
4 T. A. Cavanaugh, *Hippocrates' Oath and Asclepius' Snake: The Birth of the Medical Profession* (Oxford: Oxford University Press, 2018), 2.
5 Ibid., 84.
6 Hippocrates, *Of the Epidemics*, trans. Francis Adams, Section II, number 2. Available at http://classics.mit.edu/Hippocrates/epidemics.1.i.html.
7 The text of my talk was published as "The Physician's Vocation," *Mercator*, September 14, 2018, https://www.mercatornet.com/the-physicians-vocation.
8 "It was the Scholastics, not the Greeks, Romans, Muslims, or Chinese, who based their studies on human dissection. In fact, during classical times, the 'dignity of the human body forbade dissection,' which is why

Greco-Roman works on anatomy are so faulty. Aristotle's studies were limited entirely to animal dissections, as were those of Celsius and Galen. Human dissection was also prohibited in Islam. But, with the founding of Christian universities came a new outlook on dissection. The starting assumption was that what was unique to humans was a soul, not a body. Therefore, dissections of the human body had no theological implications. To this, two justifications were added. The first was forensic. Too many murderers escaped detection because the bodies of their victims were not subjected to a careful postmortem. The second was that adequate medical knowledge required direct observation of human anatomy. Consequently, in the thirteenth century, local officials (especially in Italian university towns) began to authorize postmortems in instances when the cause of death was uncertain. Then, late in the century, Mondino de'Luzzi (1270–1326) wrote a textbook on dissection, based on his study of two female cadavers. Subsequently, in about 1315, he performed a human dissection in front of an audience of students and faculty at the University of Bologna. From there, human dissection spread quite rapidly throughout the Italian universities—given added impetus by the calamity of the Black Death. Public dissections began in Spain in 1391, and the first one in Vienna was conducted in 1404. Nor were these rare occurrences—dissection became a customary part of anatomy classes. The 'introduction [of human dissection] in the Latin west, made without serious objection from the Church, was a momentous occurrence.'" Rodney Stark, *Bearing False Witness: Debunking Centuries of Anti-Catholic History* (West Conshohocken: Templeton Press, 2016), 142–43, Kindle.

9   See Michel Foucault, *The Birth of the Clinic: An Archeology of Medical Perception*, trans A. M. Sheridan Smith (New York: Vintage Books, 1973).
10   Jeffrey P. Bishop, *The Anticipatory Corpse: Medicine and the Care of the Dying* (Notre Dame: University of Notre Dame Press, 2011), 51.
11   Ibid.
12   Foucault, *The Birth of the Clinic*, 124–25.
13   Ibid., 125.
14   Fyodor Dostoyevsky, *Crime and Punishment*, trans. Sidney Monas (New York: Signet Classics, 2006).
15   Arthur C. Guyton and John E Hall, *Textbook of Medical Physiology*, 11th ed. (New York: W. B. Saunders, 2006), 3.
16   Claude Bernard, *An Introduction to the Study of Experimental Medicine*, trans. Henry Copley Greene (New York: Dover Publications, 1957), 82.
17   Ibid., 99.
18   Ibid.
19   Ibid., 103.

20 Iain McGilchrist, *The Matter with Things: Our Brains, Our Delusions, and the Unmaking of the World* (London: Perspectiva Press, 2021), 674. See chapter 12 for a critique of mechanistic materialism in biology and why organisms are not machines.
21 Craig Holdrege, ed., *The Dynamic Heart and Circulation*, trans. Katherine Creeger (AWSNA Publications, 2002), 12. Cited in McGilchrist, *The Matter with Things*, 690.
22 McGilchrist, *The Matter with Things*, 712.
23 Ibid.
24 Ibid, 735.

CHAPTER 3

1 Plato, *Republic*, trans. C. D. C. Reeve (Indianapolis: Hackett Publishing Company, 2004) Book III, 405d.
2 Molière, *The Imaginary Invalid*, in *The Dramatic Works of Molière*, trans. Henri Van Laun (Philadelphia: George Barrie & Sons, 1908), Act III, Scene 2, 3:239.
3 Stanton C. Pimper pimped. *JAMA*, 1989;262(17):2541–2542, doi:10.1001/jama.1989.03430170181047.
4 Ludwig Wittgenstein, *Tractatus Logico-Philosophicus*, trans. C. K. Ogden (Mineola: Dover Publications, 1999), 68.
5 David K. O'Connor, "The Names of Love," *First Things* no. 116 (October 2001): 14–15.
6 Ibid.
7 Ivan Illich, *Medical Nemesis: The Expropriation of Health*, 1st American ed. (New York: Pantheon Books, 1976), 170–71.
8 Ibid.
9 Ibid.
10 E. Richard Brown, *Rockefeller Medicine Men: Medicine and Capitalism in America* (Berkeley: University of California Press, 1979), 80–81.
11 R. Moynihan, I. Heath, and D. Henry, "Selling Sickness: The Pharmaceutical Industry and Disease Mongering," *BMJ* 324 (April 13, 2002): 886, https://doi.org/10.1136/bmj.324.7342.886.
12 Illich, *Medical Nemesis*, 106.
13 Ibid., 205, 7.

CHAPTER 4

1 Blaise Pascal, *Pensées*, trans. Roger Ariew (Indianapolis: Hackett Publishing, 2005), Fragment 165, p. 47.
2 William Shakespeare, *As You Like It*, Act 2, Scene 7.
3 "WHO Recommendations: Non-Clinical Interventions to Reduce Unnecessary Caesarean Sections," World Health Organization, October 11, 2018, https://www.who.int/publications/i/item/9789241550338.

4   Joyce A. Martin, Brady E. Hamilton, and Michelle J. K. Osterman, "Births in the United States, 2020," NCHS Data Brief, No. 418, September 2021.
5   Ibid.
6   Matthias Claudius, "Der Mensch (The Human Being)," English translation available at https://allpoetry.com/Matthias-Claudius.
7   Ibid.
8   Samuel Beckett, *Waiting for Godot: A Tragicomedy in Two Acts* (New York: Grove Press, 1954), 57.
9   *Media vita in morte sumus*, traditionally attributed to Notker the Stammerer, a ninth-century monk, and later incorporated into the Catholic liturgy and the Anglican *Book of Common Prayer*.
10 Paul Ramsey, *The Patient as Person; Explorations in Medical Ethics*, The Lyman Beecher Lectures at Yale University (New Haven: Yale University Press, 1970), 130.
11 Ernest Becker, *The Denial of Death* (New York: Free Press, 1973), 66.
12 Ira Byock, *The Four Things That Matter Most: A Book About Living* (New York: Free Press, 2004).
13 Remark made on September 19, 1777, during a conversation about the impending execution of a man named Dr. William Dodd, a clergyman convicted of forgery. James Boswell, *The Life of Samuel Johnson, LL.D.*, ed. George Birkbeck Hill and L. F. Powell, vol. 3 (Oxford: Clarendon Press, 1934), 167.
14 Job 13:15, New International Version (NIV) translation.
15 Dylan Thomas, *In Country Sleep and Other Poems* (New York: New Directions, 1952), 18.
16 Thomas Aquinas, *Summa Theologiae* (Second Part of the Second Part, Question 123, Article 4).
17 Paul Ramsey, "The Indignity of 'Death with Dignity'," *The Hastings Center Studies* 2, no. 2 (May 1974): 47–62, https://doi.org/10.2307/3527482.
18 Sherwin B. Nuland, *How We Die: Reflections on Life's Final Chapter* (New York: Random House Large Print in association with Alfred A. Knopf, 1994).
19 Blaise Pascal, *Pensées*, trans. W. F. Trotter (New York: E. P. Dutton, 1958), fragment 347, p. 100.
20 Robert Spaemann, *Persons: The Difference Between "Someone" and "Something"*, trans. Oliver O'Donovan (Oxford: Oxford University Press, 2006), 40–60.

CHAPTER 5
1   T. S. Eliot, *Four Quartets* (New York: Harcourt, Brace and Company, 1943).
2   See my article, "Dying of Despair," *First Things*, Number 275, August/September 2017.

3   Jeffrey Paul Bishop, *The Anticipatory Corpse: Medicine, Power, and the Care of the Dying* (Notre Dame: University of Notre Dame Press, 2011), chapter 6.
4   Associated Press, "Brain-Dead Virginia Woman Dies After Giving Birth; Was Kept on Life Support as Fetus Developed," August 3, 2005, https://www.9news.com/article/news/brain-dead-virginia-woman-dies-after-giving-birth-was-kept-on-life-support-as-fetus-developed/73-344702383.
5   D. Alan Shewmon, "Brain Death: A Conclusion in Search of a Justification," *Hastings Center Report* 48, suppl. 4 (November-December 2018): S18–S24, https://doi.org/10.1002/hast.947.
6   Paul Ramsey, *The Patient as Person; Explorations in Medical Ethics* (New Haven: Yale University Press, 1970), 209.
7   Harrington coined this phrase in the context of her critique of gender medicine, where healthy body parts are amputated to conform to the detached mind's desires and preferences. Mary Harrington, *Feminism Against Progress* (Washington: Regnery, 2023).
8   Bishop, *The Anticipatory Corpse*, 23.
9   Ibid., 285.
10 See David Kilgour and David Matas, "Report into Allegations of Organ Harvesting of Falun Gong Practitioners in China," July 2, 2006, updated in Bloody Harvest (2007), available at organharvestinvestigation.net; David Kilgour, David Matas, and Ethan Gutmann, "Bloody Harvest/The Slaughter: An Update," June 22, 2016, available at endtransplantabuse.org; M. P. Robertson, R. L. Hinde, and J. Lavee, "Analysis of Official Deceased Organ Donation Data Casts Doubt on the Credibility of China's Organ Transplant Reform," *BMC Medical Ethics* 20, no. 1 (November 2019): 79, https://doi.org/10.1186/s12910-019-0406-6;; M. P. Robertson and J. Lavee, "Execution by Organ Procurement: Breaching the Dead Donor Rule in China," *American Journal of Transplantation* 22, no. 4 (2022): 1011–19, https://doi.org/10.1111/ajt.16969.
11 For a helpful moral analysis of this issue, cf. Michael J. Sandel, *What Money Can't Buy: The Moral Limits of Markets*, 1st ed. (New York: Farrar, Straus and Giroux, 2012).

CHAPTER 6

1   Robert Burton, *The Anatomy of Melancholy, What It Is: With All the Kinds, Causes, Symptomes Prognostickes, and Several Cures of It* (Oxford: Printed by John Lichfield and James Short, for Henry Cripps, 1621), 13.
2   T. Padma, "Developing Countries: The Outcomes Paradox," *Nature* 508, S14–S15 (2014), https://doi.org/10.1038/508S14a.

3   National Research Council, *The Growth of Incarceration in the United States: Exploring Causes and Consequences* (Washington: The National Academies Press, 2014), https://doi.org/10.17226/18613. Half of all inmates have a mental illness or substance abuse disorder; 15 percent of state inmates are diagnosed with a psychotic disorder, according to the Department of Justice. See D. J. James and L. E. Glaze, *Mental Health Problems of Prison and Jail Inmates* (Washington: US Department of Justice, Office of Justice Programs, Bureau of Justice Statistics, 2006).
4   "Homeless Mentally Ill Facts and Figures," Mental Illness Policy Org, 2019, available at mentalillnesspolicy.org. This source aggregates data indicating that around 33 percent of homeless individuals in the US suffer from serious mental illnesses, with higher rates among the chronically homeless.

CHAPTER 7
1   William Shakespeare, *Macbeth*, ed. Barbara A. Mowat and Paul Werstine (New York: Folger Shakespeare Library, 2013), 5.3.42–46.
2   T. S. Eliot, *Four Quartets* (New York: Harcourt, Brace and Company, 1943), 19.
3   Dave Matthews, "Grey Street," track 2 on Dave Matthews Band, *Busted Stuff*, RCA Records, 2002.
4   Robert Lowell, "I.A. Richards 2. Death," lines 7–8, *History* (London: Faber and Faber, 1973), 202.
5   Walker Percy, *The Moviegoer* (New York: Vintage, 1998), 233.
6   Gerard Manley Hopkins, "The Blessed Virgin Compared to the Air We Breathe," in *The Poetical Works of Gerard Manley Hopkins*, ed. Norman H. Mackenzie (Oxford: Clarendon Press, 1990), 185.

CHAPTER 8
1   Job 5:18, Revised Standard Version (RSV) translation.
2   His real name.
3   Edmund D. Pellegrino, "The Internal Morality of Clinical Medicine: A Paradigm for the Ethics of the Helping and Healing Professions," *Journal of Medicine and Philosophy* 26, no. 6 (2001).
4   Leo Tolstoy, *Anna Karenina*, trans. Constance Garnett (New York: Modern Library, 2000), part 3, chapter 5.

CHAPTER 9
1   The Police, "King of Pain," *Synchronicity*, A&M Records, 1983.
2   George Eliot, *Middlemarch*, ed. Rosemary Ashton (London: Penguin Classics, 1994), 896.
3   Job 38:2–4, Revised Standard Version (RSV) translation.
4   Psalm 39:7–13, Revised Standard Version (RSV) translation.

5   Karl Jaspers, *Philosophy and the World: Selected Essays and Lectures* (Washington: Regnery Gateway, 1989),163.
6   Ibid., 166.
7   Ibid.
8   Ibid., 164–5.
9   Ibid., 165.
10 Ibid.
11 Ibid.
12 T. S. Eliot, *Four Quartets*, "East Coker," Part II (New York: Harcourt, Brace and Company, 1943).

CHAPTER 10

1   William Osler, *The Principles and Practice of Medicine* (New York: D. Appleton and Company, 1892). See also Jeffrey K. Aronson, "When I Use a Word . . . Listening to the Patient," *BMJ* 376 (2022): o646, https://www.bmj.com/content/376/bmj.o646.
2   Brian Kennedy, Alec Tyson, and Cary Funk, "Americans' Trust in Scientists, Other Groups Declines," Pew Research Center, February 15 2022, https://www.pewresearch.org/science/2022/02/15/americans-trust-in-scientists-other-groups-declines/.
3   "Survey on Trust in Health Care," ABIM Foundation, 2021, retrieved from https://abimfoundation.org/building-trust. See also D. B. Wolfson and "Increasing Trust in Health Care," *The American Journal of Managed Care* 27, no. 12 (December 2021): 520–22, https://doi.org/10.37765/ajmc.2021.88790.
4   Aaron Kheriaty, *The New Abnormal: The Rise of the Biomedical Security State* (Washington: Regnery Publishing, 2022).
5   The Beryl Institute and Ipsos, "PX Pulse: Consumer Perspectives on Patient Experience—Q4 2022," (Nashville: The Beryl Institute, 2022), https://www.ipsos.com/en-us/knowledge/society/Consumer-Perspectives-on-Patient-Experience-in-the-US.
6   See the Harris Poll, "The Patient Experience: Perspectives on Today's Healthcare," conducted for the American Academy of Physician Associates, May 17, 2023, https://www.aapa.org/news-central/2023/05/u-s-adults-spend-eight-hours-monthly-coordinating-healthcare-find-system-overwhelming/.
7   Paige Nong et al., "Patient-Reported Experiences of Discrimination in the US Health Care System," *JAMA Network Open* 3, no. 12 (2020): e2029650, https://pubmed.ncbi.nlm.nih.gov/33320264/.
8   See N. S. Lyons, "The China Convergence," *The Upheaval* Substack, August 3, 2023, https://theupheaval.substack.com/p/the-china-convergence.
9   See Sarah W. Fraser and Trisha Greenhalgh, "Coping with Complexity: Educating for Capability," *BMJ* 323 (October 6, 2001): 799–803, https:

//doi.org/10.1136/bmj.323.7316.799, available at https://www.ncbi.nlm.nih.gov/pmc/articles/PMC1121342/pdf/799.pdf.
10. Harvey Risch, "Plausibility but Not Science Has Dominated Public Discussions of the Covid Pandemic," Brownstone Institute, November 26, 2022, https://brownstone.org/articles/plausibility-but-not-science-has-dominated-public-discussions-of-the-covid-pandemic/.
11. Ibid.
12. Ibid.
13. See for example the Cass Review, commissioned by the National Health Service in the United Kingdom, available at https://cass.independent-review.uk/home/publications/final-report/.
14. R. K. Wadhera et al., "Quality Measure Development and Associated Spending by the Centers for Medicare & Medicaid Services," *JAMA* 323, no. 16 (April 28, 2020): 1614–16, https://doi.org/10.1001/jama.2020.1816.
15. L. P. Casalino et al., "US Physician Practices Spend More Than $15.4 Billion Annually to Report Quality Measures," *Health Affairs* 35, no. 3 (March 2016): 401–406, https://doi.org/10.1377/hlthaff.2015.1258.
16. Several review articles have failed to demonstrate that lowering cholesterol lowers the risk of heart disease, yet this remains dogma within cardiology. See for example, U. Ravnskov et al., "Lack of an Association or an Inverse Association Between Low-Density-Lipoprotein Cholesterol and Mortality in the Elderly: A Systematic Review," *BMJ Open* 6, no. 6 (June 12, 2016): e010401, https://doi.org/10.1136/bmjopen-2015-010401; U. Ravnskov et al., "LDL-C Does Not Cause Cardiovascular Disease: A Comprehensive Review of the Current Literature," *Expert Review of Clinical Pharmacology* 11, no. 10 (October 11, 2018): 959–70, https://doi.org/10.1080/17512433.2018.1519391.
17. Geoffrey Chaucer, *The Canterbury Tales*, ed. Jill Mann (London: Penguin Classics, 2005), 15–16, lines 411–44.
18. See Abraham M. Nussbaum, "Duty Hours," chap. 8 in *The Finest Traditions of My Calling: One Physician's Search for the Renewal of Medicine* (New Haven: Yale University Press, 2016).
19. See Edward Gibbon, *The History of the Decline and Fall of the Roman Empire*, 6 vols. (London: Strahan & Cadell, 1776–1789), especially Volume 1, where he discusses the attempted reforms of Diocletian.
20. See Michael Loewe, *Everyday Life in Early Imperial China During the Han Period, 202 BC–AD 220* (London: B. T. Batsford; New York: G. P. Putnam's Sons, 1968).
21. David Webster, *The Collapse of the Classic Maya Civilization* (Cambridge: Cambridge University Press, 2002).
22. See for example, John P. A. Ioannidis, "Why Most Published Research Findings Are False," *PLoS Medicine* 2, no. 8 (August 30, 2005): e124, https://doi.org/10.1371/journal.pmed.0020124. Florian Prinz, Thomas

Schlange, and Khusru Asadullah, "Believe It or Not: How Much Can We Rely on Published Data on Potential Drug Targets?," *Nature Reviews Drug Discovery* 10, no. 9 (August 31, 2011): 712, https://doi.org/10.1038/nrd3439-c1; C. Glenn Begley and Lee M. Ellis, "Raise Standards for Preclinical Cancer Research," *Nature* 483 (2012): 531–33, https://doi.org/10.1038/483531a; Open Science Collaboration, "Estimating the Reproducibility of Psychological Science," *Science* 349, no. 6251 (August 28, 2015): aac4716, https://doi.org/10.1126/science.aac4716.
23 Illich, *Medical Nemesis*, 3.
24 Ibid., 4.
25 Ibid.
26 Ibid., 6.
27 Ibid., 7.
28 Cited in Ibid., 6.
29 See references in Ibid., 16.
30 Ibid., 17–20.
31 Ibid., 11.
32 See Lauren Weber and Anna Maria Barry-Jester, "Over Half of States Have Rolled Back Public Health Powers in Pandemic," KFF Health News, 2021, retrieved from kffhealthnews.org.
33 Illich, *Medical Nemesis*, 29–30.
34 Ibid., 62.
35 J. O'Neill, "Tackling Drug-Resistant Infections Globally: Final Report and Recommendations," Review on Antimicrobial Resistance, May 2016, available at: https://amr-review.org/. This report highlights how antibiotics' short treatment duration (e.g., a one-time or week-long course) yields lower returns compared to drugs for chronic diseases like diabetes or hypertension, which generate recurring revenue. It notes that the net present value (NPV) of a new antibiotic is often negative (estimated at -$50 million), while a drug for a musculoskeletal condition might reach +$1.15 billion. See also Carl Nathan and Frederick M. Goldberg, "The Profit Problem in Antibiotic R&D," *Nature Reviews Drug Discovery* 4 (2005): 887–91, https://doi.org/10.1038/nrd1878; World Health Organization, "Lack of New Antibiotics Threatens Global Efforts to Contain Drug-Resistant Infections," 2020, retrieved from https://www.who.int/news/item/17-01-2020-lack-of-new-antibiotics-threatens-global-efforts-to-contain-drug-resistant-infections; Benjamin Plackett, "Why Big Pharma Has Abandoned Antibiotics," *Nature* 586, no. S50–52 (October 2020), https://doi.org/10.1038/d41586-020-02884-3.
36 In the US, the American Cancer Society (ACS) reported 1.9 million new cases in 2022, ticking up to over 2 million in 2023. By 2024, they estimated 2,001,140 new cases. This upward trend isn't just about more people

or better detection; for some cancers, it's a real increase. See American Cancer Society, "Cancer Facts & Figures 2022," "Cancer Facts & Figures 2023," and "Cancer Facts & Figures 2024" at cancer.org. Six of the top ten cancers—breast, prostate, endometrial, pancreatic, kidney, and melanoma—are showing higher incidence, often linked to lifestyle shifts like rising obesity. See R. L. Siegel et al., "Cancer Statistics, 2024," *CA: A Cancer Journal for Clinicians* 74, no. 1 (January 2024): 12–49, https://doi.org/10.3322/caac.21820. Younger adults are a particular concern. Early-onset cancers (under age 50) have spiked globally—up nearly 80 percent in cases from 1990 to 2019. See J. Zhao et al., "Global Trends in Incidence, Death, Burden and Risk Factors of Early-Onset Cancer From 1990 to 2019," *BMJ Oncology* 2, no. 1 (September 2023): e000049, https://bmjoncology.bmj.com/content/2/1/e000049.

37 To mention just one example among many, a 2019 study found that 24 percent of new antidepressant prescriptions for elderly patients were potentially overprescribed. These were mostly newer drugs like SSRIs and SNRIs, handed out for vague "non-specific psychiatric symptoms" or subthreshold conditions (e.g., adjustment disorders, bereavement) rather than clear-cut diagnoses like major depression. Overprescription was tied to nursing home stays, more comorbidities, and prescriptions via phone or email—hinting at sloppy, non-face-to-face decision-making. This suggests overprescribing often occurs when clinical complexity or convenience trumps rigorous assessment. See T. G. Rhee, J. C. Schommer, B. D. Capistrant, R. L. Hadsall, and D. L. Uden, "Potentially Inappropriate Antidepressant Prescriptions Among Older Adults in Office-Based Outpatient Settings: National Trends from 2002 to 2012," *Adm Policy Ment Health* 45, no. 2 (March 2018): 224–35, doi: 10.1007/s10488-017-0817-y. PMID: 28730279. Similarly, a 2011 study found that between 1996 and 2007, the proportion of antidepressant prescriptions without a psychiatric diagnosis jumped from 60 percent to 73 percent. By 2007, over 10 percent of US adults were on antidepressants, yet many lacked documented mental health conditions. This points to a trend of "off-label" or casual prescribing, possibly fueled by direct-to-consumer ads or time-pressed primary care docs leaning on pills over therapy. See R. Mojtabai and M. Olfson, "National Trends in Psychotropic Medication Polypharmacy in Office-Based Psychiatry," *Archives of General Psychiatry* 67, no. 1 (January 2010): 26–36, https://doi.org/10.1001/archgenpsychiatry.2009.175.

38 Munira Z. Gunja et al. "U.S. Health Care from a Global Perspective, 2022: Accelerating Spending, Worsening Outcomes," The Commonwealth Fund, January 31, 2023, https://www.commonwealthfund.org/publications/issue-briefs/2023/jan/us-health-care-global-perspective-2022.

39 Ibid.

40 For more on Lewis Mumford's concept of the megamachine, a machine made of human parts, see my summary in Kheriaty, *The New Abnormal*, 18–27.
41 Illich, *Medical Nemesis*, 274–5.
42 Ibid., 11.
43 Ibid., 271.

CHAPTER 11
1 William Osler, "The Army Surgeon," *The Medical News* 64, no. 19 (May 12, 1894): 549–552.
2 The concept of a parallel polis was elaborated by the Czech dissident Václav Benda, who along with Václav Havel (later the first president of the Czech Republic following the fall of communism) and other collaborators opposed the Soviet Communist regime in the 1970s. See Benda's essay on the parallel polis in Václav Benda, *The Long Night of the Watchman: Essays by Václav Benda, 1977–1989*, ed. F. Flagg Taylor IV (South Bend: St. Augustine's Press, 2017).
3 Aaron Kheriaty, "Rebellion, Not Retreat," *The American Mind*, June 27, 2023, https://americanmind.org/salvo/rebellion-not-retreat/.
4 "2024 Direct Primary Care," Data Brief, American Academy of Family Physicians, 2023, https://www.aafp.org/about/policies/all/direct-primary-care.html. See also Direct Primary Care Coalition, "DPC Practice Map and Legislative Updates," https://www.aafp.org/dam/AAFP/documents/practice_management/direct-primary-care-2024-data-brief.pdf. See also Direct Primary Care Coalition at https://www.dpcare.org.
5 P. M. Eskew, et al., "Economic Viability of Direct Primary Care: A Comparative Analysis with Fee-for-Service Models," *Journal of General Internal Medicine*, 39(5), 795–801, 2024, DOI: 10.1007/s11606-023-08524-3. This study simulates a 500-patient DPC practice at $75/month against FFS benchmarks. See also L. P. Casalino et al., "US Physician Practices Spend More Than $15.4 Billion Annually to Report Quality Measures," *Health Affairs* 35, no. 3 (March 2016): 401–6, https://doi.org/10.1377/hlthaff.2015.1258.
6 D. N. Bryan, "Benefits of Direct Primary Care in Improving Quality and Reducing Costs of Healthcare," Mercatus Center, January 19, 2021, https://www.mercatus.org/research/state-testimonies/benefits-direct-primary-care-improving-quality-and-reducing-costs.
7 J. Wu et al., "The Cost-Effectiveness Analysis of the New Rural Cooperative Medical Scheme in China," *PLOS ONE* 13, no. 12 (December 2018): e0208297, https://doi.org/10.1371/journal.pone.0208297. See also Congressional Budget Office, "Cost Estimate for America's Healthy Future Act of 2009," Letter to Senator Max Baucus, October 7, 2009, https://www.cbo.gov/publication/41335.

8   Paul Starr, *The Social Transformation of American Medicine: The Rise of a Sovereign Profession and the Making of a Vast Industry* (New York: Basic Books, 1982), 32.
9   Cited in ibid.
10 Starr, *The Social Transformation of American Medicine*, 33.
11 Cited in ibid.
12 Starr, *The Social Transformation of American Medicine*, 34.
13 For more information, including information on how to start a new chapter, go to https://hippsoc.org.
14 See for example, Victor Davis Hanson, John Heath, and Bruce S. Thornton, *Bonfire of the Humanities: Rescuing the Classics in an Impoverished Age* (Wilmington: ISI Books, 2001). See also Allan Bloom's well-known critique in his bestselling book *The Closing of the American Mind: How Higher Education Has Failed Democracy and Impoverished the Souls of Today's Students* (New York: Simon & Schuster, 1987).
15 Karl Jaspers, *Philosophy and the World: Selected Essays and Lectures* (Washington: Regnery Gateway, 1989), 163.
16 Walker Percy, *Signposts in a Strange Land* (New York: Farrar, Straus & Giroux, 1991), 272.

CONCLUSION
1   T. S. Eliot, *Four Quartets* (New York: Harcourt, Brace and Company, 1943).
2   Thomas Nagel, "What Is It Like to Be a Bat?," *The Philosophical Review* 83, no. 4 (October 1974): 435–50, https://doi.org/10.2307/2183914.
3   Francis W. Peabody, "The Care of the Patient," *Journal of American College Health* 33, no. 5 (1985): 210–16, https://doi.org/10.1080/07448481.1985.9939607.
4   Leonard Cohen, "Hallelujah," *Various Positions*, Columbia Records, 1984.
5   Phillip Phillips, "Home," *The World from the Side of the Moon*, Interscope Records, 2012.